ETHICAL ISSUES IN HOME HEALTH CARE

ETHICAL ISSUES IN HOME HEALTH CARE

By

ROSALIND EKMAN LADD, Ph.D.

Wheaton College
Norton, Massachusetts

LYNN PASQUERELLA, Ph.D.

University of Rhode Island
Kingston, Rhode Island

SHERI SMITH, Ph.D.

Rhode Island College
Providence, Rhode Island

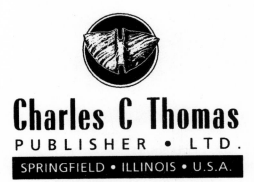

Charles C Thomas
PUBLISHER • LTD.
SPRINGFIELD • ILLINOIS • U.S.A.

Published and Distributed Throughout the World by

CHARLES C THOMAS • PUBLISHER, LTD.
2600 South First Street
Springfield, Illinois 62704

ISBN 0-398-07283-3 (hard)
ISBN 0-398-07284-1 (paper)

Library of Congress Catalog Card Number: 2002018926

With THOMAS BOOKS *careful attention is given to all details of man-
ufacturing and design. It is the Publisher's desire to present books that are satisfactory as to their physical qualities and artistic possibilities and appropriate for their particular use.* THOMAS BOOKS *will be true to those laws
of quality that assure a good name and good will.*

Printed in the United States of America
CR-R-3

Library of Congress Cataloging-in-Publication Data

Ladd, Rosalind Ekman.
   Ethical issues in home health care / by Rosalind Ekman Ladd,
Lynn Pasquerella, Sheri Smith
      p.   cm.
   Includes bibliographical references and index.
   ISBN 0-398-07283-3 -- ISBN 0-398-07284-1 (pbk.)
    1. Home care services--Moral and ethical aspects. 2. Home nursing--Moral
and ethical aspects. 3. Nursing ethics. I. Pasquerella, Lynn. II. Smith, Sheri,
Ph.D. III. Title

RA645.3 .L33 2002
174'.2--dc21
                                                                    2002018926

For the many nurses who generously shared their stories with us.
– *R.E.L. and S.L.S.*

For my parents Patricia and Francis, who first taught me about caring, and my sons Pierce and Spencer, from whom I continue to learn daily. – *L.P.*

PREFACE

This book lets us listen to the voices of home health care nurses as they pose the ethical questions they encounter in their work. The cases presented in each chapter are fictionalized situations based on interviews conducted with home health care nurses in both hospital-sponsored and private agencies, in hospices, and in urban and rural settings. We have attempted to avoid the use of gendered pronouns, except in the discussion of cases, where their use reflects the fact that the majority of nurses in home health care are women.

Home health care is an increasingly important venue for nursing, as advances in medical technology and cost-containing measures shift the ill population from hospital to home. In this practice setting, nurses voice ethical concerns that are importantly different from the ethical questions most common in hospital nursing practice. Nursing literature frequently addresses ethical issues, but little attention has been paid to the special circumstances of home health care and the fact that this kind of nursing requires different strategies for effective ethical responses.

Each chapter of this book is devoted to one of the main areas of concern for home health care nurses. Focusing on specific cases, it offers analysis and discussion of the ethical issues, cites legal requirements where relevant, and summarizes ethical criteria and practical strategies. The discussion of these cases is not intended to be comprehensive, but to serve as a useful stimulus for further, indepth discussion of the issues. The initial cases from each chapter are discussed in the concluding chapter.

The goal is for the reader to develop a keen sensitivity to ethical questions and skill in the critical thinking process that leads to careful, reasoned decisions about what to do. Reflection on the issues and attention to the reasoning process can aid nurses, clients, families, and other caregivers as they confront the emotion-laden decisions of home health care ethics.

ACKNOWLEDGMENTS

We are indebted to many individuals who both enriched our work and made it possible, beginning with the nurses who shared their stories with us and the agencies that provided us with access. Special recognition should be given to the Rhode Island State Nurses Association and to the nursing faculty at Rhode Island College and the University of Rhode Island. Several nursing scholars made unique contributions. From the project's inception, Mary E. Byrd's inspiration and advice have proven instrumental in the design and evolution of our research and the development of this book. Joanne Costello, M.P.H., M.N., R.N., C.S., and Jane Williams, Ph.D., R.N., have also contributed enormously by offering insights into the nature of nursing practice in the home health care context. We are also grateful to Trudy C. Mulvey, M.S.N., R.N., C.S., and Maureen Newman, Ph.D., R.N., C.S. for their insights about home health care nursing. Professor Byrd, Ph.D., R.N., C.S. Professor Costello, and Professor Williams, together with Carol Reagan Shelton, Ph.D., R.N., and Patricia A. Thomas, Ph.D., R.N.C., assisted us by reading and commenting on drafts of chapters. Their efforts improved the book considerably, though any mistakes are, of course, our own. In addition, members of the planning committee, Virginia Tougas Conway, R.N., B.S., Mary Ellen M. Januario, R.N., Pamela L. McCue, M.S.N., R.N., and participants at the home health care conference "How Far Should We Go? Practical Approaches to Ethical Dilemmas: Managed Care, Noncompliance and End of Life Decisions" provided valuable feedback on many of the case studies we developed.

We also appreciate the support of friends, colleagues, and family members, whose presence, conversations, and encouragement were indispensable to us during the process of research and writing. We hope they know the extent of our gratitude.

CONTENTS

ETHICAL ISSUES IN HOME HEALTH CARE

Chapter 1

INTRODUCTION:
ETHICAL DECISION MAKING

I have a client who is dying at home. Her family has been wonderful with her. Her two sisters are taking care of her, and they are with her all the time. She told me they pray together. She just seems so peaceful, even though her condition is deteriorating. Recently she obstructed, but she said she didn't want a colostomy. She didn't think her sisters could deal with it. **Should I support her decision to spare her family?**

General Issues

- **What is ethics?**
- **How should claims about rights be used in making ethical decisions?**
- **What role should consequences have in ethical decision making?**
- **What other factors should be considered?**

The nurse in this case faces a classic ethical dilemma, that is, a conflict between two moral ideals. One ideal holds that nurses should respect a client's right to make decisions, but here that ideal conflicts with the responsibility nurses also have to promote a client's health and well-being. The decision the nurse must make in this situation is different from the clinical decisions she confronts every day, for this involves the kind of question that goes beyond facts. The uncertainty about what it is right to do cannot be resolved by gathering more factual information or even through further assessment of a client's clinical condition. Instead, answering ethical questions requires skill in identifying the significant moral factors in a situation and then reasoning to a conclusion about the best course of action.

3

This case illustrates three important features of the special challenges home health care nurses face when ethical conflicts arise: First, although they are part of an interdisciplinary team, home health care nurses are usually the only professionals in the home when a decision must be made. Second, the home setting itself may be the source of moral concerns, for example, if obstacles exist that prevent ideal nursing interventions on behalf of a client. Third, though their primary responsibility is to care for clients, nurses must also respond to concerns about family members or others who are caregivers. As a result, the ethical dilemmas nurses face in home health care may be complex and, in some instances, unique to the home setting.

Ideally, home health care nurses will be adept at thinking through solutions to ethical problems, without the benefit of immediate advice from professional colleagues, and they will be able to assist clients and families in understanding and coping with difficult decisions. These skills can be developed through thoughtful reflection on ethics and ethical decision making.

WHAT IS ETHICS?

Ethics involves critical reflection on fundamental moral beliefs, that is, beliefs about how to live, what has meaning and value, and what is morally right to do. The ultimate goal of careful reflection on these issues is a decision or a claim about morality that is thoughtful and well supported by reasons. Thus, reasonable answers to these moral questions and good ethical decisions will be the result of critical thinking.

Laws and nursing codes of ethics offer legal standards and moral ideals for the practice of nursing, but they cannot substitute for ongoing critical thinking about ethical issues. Laws, for example, are not very helpful in determining what is ethically right to do, because they state legal standards that are often vague and which need to be interpreted. Because legal standards are also subject to ethical evaluation, the laws themselves could possibly be judged immoral. Moreover, many of the circumstances that present ethical dilemmas are not covered by the law. For these reasons, ethics requires going beyond the view known as legalism, the idea that right and wrong are fully determined by the legal requirements that apply to a situation.

Nursing codes of ethics outline the basic moral principles that should guide the professional practice of nursing and serve to inspire moral ideals for practice. However, codes of ethics, like laws, generally offer vague statements that require interpretation in a specific case to determine what to do. According to the American Nurses Association Code of Ethics, for example, a nurse's primary commitment is to the health, safety, and rights of the patient. The dilemma that arises when these moral requirements conflict is well illustrated in the situation described earlier. Referring to the code of ethics clearly does not resolve that dilemma. Instead, a resolution calls for weighing these requirements against each other to determine what should be done.

Finally, though religions are a common source of basic ethical principles, neither ethical thinking nor ethical behavior requires a basis in a religion or in religious beliefs. What good ethical thinking does require is reflection on the reasons that support a decision.

However, even careful ethical reasoning will not produce judgments that are beyond dispute or challenge. Some disputes can be resolved by identifying and analyzing the reasons that support different views, if individuals can agree that some reasons are more compelling. Other disagreements, though, stem from differences in values. Reasonable people may disagree about important values or the relevance of specific moral considerations and thus arrive at different answers to ethical questions. The practical issue of what to do when disagreements persist can sometimes be resolved if it can be determined who has the authority to make the final decision.

TRADITIONAL ETHICS

Each traditional ethical theory consists of a set of moral values and principles. These are the basis for identifying the features of a situation that are morally significant and thus provide the rationale for a decision about what is right to do. There are two commonly used approaches to ethical decision making, one that specifies rights and a second that identifies consequences as the crucial factors to consider. Both approaches are reflected in public policy, professional decisions, and everyday choices.

Oftentimes there is a conflict between family members and the clients themselves. I have a situation where the client has a cancer diagnosis and was discharged home with home health care. Her daughter insists on making all the
medical decisions for her mother, and the physicians go along with this. The
plan is to transfer the client into a hospice program. But no one knows what
the client wants, because no one has asked her. **Doesn't she have a right to
make these decisions herself?**

The rights-based approach to making ethical decisions is based on
the claim that specific actions are required because of the moral and
legal rights of individuals. This method can be applied by asking these
questions: (1) What are the moral and legal rights of each person
involved? and (2) How should those rights be weighted? In cases of
conflict, which rights take precedence?

This method can be used to answer the questions raised by the previous case. Unless the client is incompetent, or she has asked her
daughter to make these decisions, the client in this case has the fundamental right to make her own decisions about her care. This places
the responsibility on others to consult her and to abide by her wishes.
At the same time, the family care-givers have rights that should also be
considered. For example, the client's daughter has the right to make
her own decisions about matters affecting her, such as whether her
mother will live with her. The client's right to decide may conflict with
her daughter's rights, for example, if she were to insist on staying with
her daughter against her daughter's wishes. If there is a conflict
between the rights of those involved, those rights must be weighted to
determine which takes precedence. Negotiation and compromise may
sometimes be necessary to resolve a conflict between rights.

I have a client who is a very frail eighty-year-old. I can't get him institutionalized because he refuses. There is no medical reason to keep him on service, but
I am concerned about him. He is really unsafe living at home alone. I could
say he needs physical therapy. **Should I do that?**

A second approach to ethical decision making is based on an evaluation of the consequences of possible actions, that is, the costs and benefits. This method can be applied by asking these questions: (1) What
are the consequences, positive and negative, of each alternative? and
(2) Which alternative offers the most benefit and the least cost overall?
Which consequences should be given the most weight?

All consequences, both short-term and long-term, should be considered when the results of a proposed course of action are evaluated. In this case, the short-term consequences of claiming the client needs physical therapy appear to be positive. Because the client will be able to stay on service, he will have the advantage of visits from a professional caregiver who can check on him, and he may be safer than he would be if discharged from service. However, the long-term negative consequences outweigh these positive results. For example, a nurse's deception, even though well-intentioned, could damage her relationship with her agency and with the other health care professionals involved. Her relationship with her client may also be jeopardized if he begins to question her trustworthiness, in light of her dishonesty on his behalf. In the final analysis, the nurse's deception cannot be justified by appealing to the results.

BEYOND TRADITIONAL ETHICS

Traditional methods are not always successful in resolving ethical dilemmas, because appeals to rights and consequences may yield conflicting answers. This book develops an approach to ethical reasoning that goes beyond traditional theories. This new approach reflects the special insights discovered by examining the nurse-client-family relationship as it occurs in the practice of home health care nursing. Careful analysis reveals that additional moral factors are relevant when ethical issues in home health care are addressed: Ethical decisions should be specific to the particular context in which the issue arises, sensitive to the relationships of those involved, and attentive to issues about character.

My client is an elderly man with congestive heart failure who has intractable pain. He has chronic severe back pain, a fracture of his ankle, and arthritis. He is on several medications. His wife is having trouble coping with all of this. She is exhausted most of the time. The biggest problem is that he is on opiates, as needed, for pain control. It is expecting a lot from her to have her figure out when he needs opiates. Even though this might be the best schedule for pain control, I'd like to recommend that the physician reconsider this. **Under the circumstances, would it be wrong to recommend less than what is optimum for pain management?**

According to traditional theories, general moral principles apply universally. That is, what is right for one person to do is right for everyone. This traditional approach, however, fails to take account of the context, in other words, the details of each person's situation and the complexity and subtlety of human emotions and relationships. In practice, ethics requires close attention to the dilemmas of particular individuals in particular situations. Thus, though it is true that cases that are alike should be treated alike, good judgment requires knowing when cases are different in relevant ways. Ethical decision making in real life involves more careful thinking about the context in which ethical issues arise than traditional theories suggest.

The preceding case illustrates the importance of context when there are ethical issues about client care. On the whole, the best schedule for pain medication should be implemented in every case. If this client were hospitalized, nurses would be able to administer opiates as needed to control his pain. However, in this particular situation, the client must depend on his elderly wife to decide that he needs opiates. When the details of the client's situation are considered, the nurse appears to be justified in recommending a change in medications, even though it is not the "best" schedule for pain control.

> We had one case—a Japanese woman. She stayed in bed, drank tea, refused to eat. She stopped eating because she was very ill and did not want to be a burden to her family. She told me it was her time. **Would it be wrong for me to accept her decision to stop eating?**

The culture of American individualism depicts individuals as isolated, independent selves making decisions only for themselves. This picture, however, does not fit the reality of the lives of most people, especially the lives of sick people in need of care. Although each client has a distinct personality, history, desire, and emotion, clients are also relatives, employees, neighbors, or friends. Each person is a self involved in relationships that are valuable and that contribute substantially to who someone is as a person.

Because relationships are so important in human lives, everyday morality recognizes that people have unique obligations that single out certain people for special treatment. These obligations supersede the moral ideal to treat all people impartially as equals. Husbands and wives, for example, have specific obligations to care for each other when they are ill—obligations that they do not have to strangers. Consequently, individuals' relationships, the duties that stem from their relationships, and the consequences actions have for relationships are crucial factors to consider when addressing ethical issues.

The client's desire to avoid burdening her family with her care is extremely meaningful in this case. Because the effects on her family are more important to her than any possible consequences for herself, this client has decided to sacrifice her interests to maintain a good relationship with her family as long as possible. It would be appropriate to address these issues about her relationships with her, but if she is clear that she wishes to make this sacrifice, that decision should be respected.

> I did something the other day that still bothers me. One of my clients is a man with Amyotrophic Lateral Sclerosis. He asked me a question about his future with ALS just as I was ready to leave. I'm usually empathetic, but I felt I didn't have the time to deal with this then. So I gave him a quick answer without giving him a chance to talk. I didn't live up to my own expectations and ideals. **Does that mean I am not a good nurse?**

Moral concerns sometimes revolve around basic issues about character. Having a good character involves more than just doing the right thing. It involves caring about what kind of person one is, being committed to developing the traits of a good person, and trying to do the right thing in the right way. While answering a client's question honestly is the right thing to do, for example, the honest answer should also be delivered in a compassionate way that shows respect for a client's concerns.

The nurse in this instance was not able to give as much time to addressing the client's worries as she believes she should ideally do. Her commitment to being a good nurse is reflected in her distress about her abrupt answer. In the final analysis, nurses like this one who strive to develop model personal characteristics, in addition to the technical skills required in professional nursing, demonstrate their essential good character.

Good ethical decision making in the home health care context should go beyond traditional ethics to address the particular circumstances of the client, the client's relationships, and issues about character. These factors should inform an evaluation of the rights and consequences that are relevant to a decision.

ETHICAL CRITERIA

• To apply the rights–based approach ask the following questions:

    1. What are the moral and legal rights of individuals?
    2. If there is a conflict, which rights take precedence?

• To apply an approach based on consequences, ask:

    1. What are the costs and benefits for each person?
    2. Which consequences should be given the most weight?
    3. Which alternative is the best for everyone overall?

• Questions about rights and consequences must be asked in ways that are specific to context, sensitive to relationships, and focused on character:

    1. Which features of the particular situation are significant?
    2. Are there personal relationships, obligations, and responsibilities that should be considered?
    3. What does this decision reveal about personal character?

Chapter 2

CLIENTS' DECISIONS, NURSES' DILEMMAS

One of my clients decided to live with his daughter so she could take care of him. The problem is he is supposed to be on oxygen all the time. His daughter doesn't want him on oxygen; she doesn't want her father to be sick. He needs a walker; his daughter tries to get him to walk without using the walker. I talked to her until I was blue in the face. I said, "You know he needs this." She is in denial. She said, "He's getting better." He lets her tell him what to do. He seems to be risking his health but he wants to stay with his daughter. **I have to let him make these decisions for himself, don't I?**

General Issues

- **Who should make decisions for clients?**
- **What is the role of the nurse if client safety is threatened?**
- **How should decisions be made for incompetent clients and children?**
- **When, if ever, may information be withheld?**

INTRODUCTION

Nurses will sometimes face ethical dilemmas about the decisions of hospitalized clients, for example, if they make decisions that risk their well-being. In the hospital setting, though, the decisions clients can make are usually restricted to choosing to accept or reject treatments. The impact of their poor judgment in these circumstances is generally limited to the consequences of treatment choices. Concerns about clients' decisions substantially broaden, however, when clients are cared for at home, where the range of decisions clients can make

11

extends from treatment choices to choices about whether to live alone or with someone else, how to run their homes, and how to manage their lives. Clients may decide to live with someone who neglects them, or even someone who is frankly dangerous, or take other risks with their own health and well-being. Consequently, the dangers of the poor decisions that clients make are amplified in the home setting.

Concerns about the safety of the setting are heightened, too, when clients are cared for in their own homes, which can harbor the sort of risks that would not exist in a hospital. The physical environment may be basically unsafe, for example, if there is substandard heating and electricity or a home lacks adequate sanitation. Clients themselves may be unable or unwilling to maintain basic standards of cleanliness. When these kinds of conditions exist, important doubts arise about whether a client should receive nursing care at home, rather than in an institution. Such concerns about clients' decisions are the source of confounding dilemmas for nurses in home health care.

WHO SHOULD MAKE DECISIONS FOR CLIENTS?

There are elderly people who are trying so hard to live at home. I'm dealing now with an elderly woman who has Parkinson's and osteoporosis. She ambulates by holding on to the furniture. I'm afraid she's going to get hurt. But when I said, "I hope you won't fall," she told me, "I'd rather take the chance I'll break a hip. It's better than going to a nursing home." **Should I respect her decision, even though I'm not comfortable with the risks she's taking?**

For nurses, clients' decisions can create a serious conflict between the basic requirement of respect for individuals' informed choices and concern for a client's well-being when those choices demonstrate poor judgment. Respect for informed decisions is required because all rational, that is, competent adults have the right to self-determination. This means that they have the right to make decisions for their lives, based on their own ideas and values. Clients thus have the right to make decisions about medical treatment, a moral right reflected in the legal requirement of informed consent. The critical challenge is to distinguish competent, though unwise choices from decisions that are not informed or not voluntary, which should be questioned.

When a competent client makes a decision that is free, deliberate, and informed, that decision must be respected. Concern for a client's well-being, that is, does not justify intervention. Thus, unless there is evidence that the client in this case is incompetent, she has the right to make the choice to continue to live alone, even though she runs the risk of incurring a serious injury. In order to respect that right and at the same time promote her safety, the nurse should try to ensure that the client understands her situation by clearly identifying the risks involved and discussing the likelihood and severity of the possible injuries risked. She should also discuss the possibility that incurring future injuries could ultimately lead to placement in a nursing home. Finally, the nurse should review with the client any steps she could take to make the home environment safer.

Nurses should document their efforts to identify risks and to communicate those risks to their clients, attempts to assist clients in making an environment safer, and efforts to find creative solutions to safety problems. Without this documentation, a nurse may be liable to disciplinary action and legal consequences if a client subsequently suffers harm.

WHEN A COMPETENT CLIENT'S SAFETY IS THREATENED

I have a new client, a young man who is a paraplegic following a car accident. He has a very positive, almost euphoric attitude. He told me he is not going to let this condition define his life. His wife is just as optimistic as he is. In fact, she just accepted a promotion, which means she'll be spending more time away from home. He encouraged her to take the promotion and assured her he could take care of himself. Of course, he can't take care of himself. When I got there yesterday, I found him on the floor. He fell and couldn't get up. I think his optimism is dangerous. **How can I make sure that I fulfill my responsibilities to keep the client safe?**

The client's own optimism may constitute a danger of sorts, if he does not correctly identify or accept the risks that are involved in trying to care for himself at home. Here the facts of the client's particular situation should be considered in assessing the risks and the options available, and the ethically appropriate response to his decisions. Particular facts about the client's home, the number of hours he is left alone, and the actions he can take if he needs assistance while his wife is out of the house, will inform the possible solutions a nurse could propose to the client. A consideration of these particular facts is also essential to determining whether the client has made an informed decision to remain in home health care under these circumstances. The nurse should focus renewed efforts on educating him about the risks of his situation, documenting her actions and her discussions with him. In that way she can meet her responsibilities to safeguard the client and respect his informed decisions.

The client's relationship to his wife is also a significant aspect of this case. His optimism may be an attempt to assure his wife that he does not need additional care and attention from her. He may be trying to protect his wife from the reality of his situation, or he may wish to ensure that she does not forfeit a career opportunity that is important to her. He could also be concerned about her reaction if he admits the true state of his health. The risks to his own safety are perhaps far less important to him than the consequences for his relationship to his wife. These consequences should be part of determining what would be right to do in this situation.

Accordingly, a nurse could encourage him to discuss these issues with his wife or ask for his permission to talk to her about his safety. Ultimately, however, if the client is competent and informed, he has the right to determine whether his wife is consulted about this, and he has the right to decide that he will continue to plan his life on the basis of his positive thinking, despite the dangers involved.

> I have a case where the client is a woman with kidney disease; she gets dialysis three times a week. I am seeing her for daily wound care. Her son moved in to take care of her. That's a joke. He has a history of alcohol abuse. He is often drunk when I arrive. I think he's neglecting her, but when I tried to talk to her about it, she said he takes good care of her. **Should I do something more to protect this woman from her own son?**

In some cases, like this one, the threats to a client's safety and well-being arise from the very people who are part of a network of significant relationships. Yet, an individual's right to make her own decisions includes the right to decide to live with family members or friends who act in ways that endanger her. As long as she is rational and competent, she can choose to have her son stay with her, even if it is not in her best interest as others would see it. The client may value her son's companionship above her own comfort, or she may wish to sacrifice her own well-being for the benefit of her son. In the absence of any clear evidence of neglect or abuse by the son, the actions a nurse would be justified in taking to protect this client are limited. She could initiate conversations with the client to explore her feelings about these issues and to assure herself that this client is making thoughtful and informed decisions. In any event, she should continue to observe the situation closely and to document carefully. Unfortunately, she will only be able to continue to monitor the situation as long as the client has skilled nursing needs which justify keeping her on service. At the first sign of abuse, the nurse must make a report to the proper authorities. Failure to report elder abuse carries various penalties, dependent on specific state statutes. In several states, the nurse would be charged with a misdemeanor and have fines imposed ranging from hundreds to thousands of dollars. In many of these states, the nurse would be subject to licensing penalties as well.

> One of my clients is on oxygen. He lives with his daughter and her boyfriend, who is a chain-smoker. The boyfriend just lost his job, so he just hangs out at the house, smoking one cigarette after another. I tried to tell both of them that no one should be smoking near my client because of the oxygen. The client doesn't seem concerned and told me to quit nagging. **Is there something else I should be doing to protect my client's safety, even though he doesn't want me to do that?**

Because of their expertise, nurses, physicians, and other health care professionals may believe that they are justified in restricting clients' rights to self-determination, for their own good. This view is called "paternalism." Paternalism would support actions to secure a client's safety, even against his own wishes. When serious safety issues arise in the home setting, paternalism may seem justified, despite the fact that it conflicts with the moral requirement to respect client self-determination.

Paternalism is clearly justified if a client is not competent, for incompetent clients should be protected from the consequences of their unwise decisions. Judging someone's competence, however, can be difficult. Strictly speaking, incompetence must be decided by a court, though in medical settings informal determinations of incompetency are often made. A legal determination of incompetence involves an assessment of orientation to time and place, ability to recognize the consequences of actions, ability to put things into logical order, and ability to make choices. If individuals are not incompetent in any of these basic ways, they are free to make decisions as unwise or risky or idiosyncratic as they please. Individuals cannot be judged incompetent simply because they make decisions that others consider unwise.

Paternalism may also be justified if a person's decision is either uninformed or involuntary. For that reason it is worth exploring why this client continues to put himself at risk. He may not clearly understand the risks involved or he may be afraid to complain about the smoking. Perhaps he fears that his daughter will become angry or that she will evict him from her house. If that is indeed his reason for accepting the risks associated with smoking in the house, then his choice may not be free and uncoerced. Intervention in that case would be justified. However, if this client is competent, and his decision is informed and voluntary, further intervention is not justified. He has the right to choose the circumstances in which he will live, no matter how dangerous.

> There are often safety concerns with elderly clients who live alone and refuse placement. They may not be legally incompetent, but they're not able to manage. I have a client who has psychiatric problems. He lives in a high-rise. He refuses to leave the apartment, refuses to go to a nursing home, but he is not safe alone. I'm trying to keep him safe by doing everything but moving in with him. I'm concerned that he will leave the stove on or that he will smoke and start a fire. **What am I justified in doing when a client demonstrates poor judgment?**

This is a difficult but not atypical situation. This client has begun to show signs of very poor judgment, but he is not incompetent. He is still alert and clear about his own wishes. However, his situation is increasingly dangerous, both to himself and to others. If he leaves the gas burner on and starts a fire, others will suffer the consequences, too. Although his power to make decisions concerning things that affect only himself must be respected in ordinary circumstances, the risk here also involves others. This consequently is a situation where intervention is justified, on the grounds that it is required for the benefit of others who could be affected by his poor judgment. In a case like this nurses should contact their supervisor about their concerns and initiate appropriate interventions.

MAKING DECISIONS FOR INCOMPETENT CLIENTS

I have a situation with a client who has Alzheimer's. His wife is trying to take care of him at home, but she really can't handle him. Yesterday when I got there, he was in the tub, just sitting there. He'd been in the tub for two days. He couldn't get out, so she covered him with a blanket and brought him his meals. She didn't call the rescue because she was afraid she wouldn't be able to keep him at home any more. **How far should I go to ensure the safety of a client who has been declared incompetent?**

Decisions for incompetent adults are usually made by the next of kin or a close friend on the basis of substituted judgment and authenticity. The standard of substituted judgment requires that the decision maker decide on the basis of what the client would have wanted if competent. The client's spoken wishes and the values expressed to others thus provide guidelines for surrogate decision makers. The goal is an authentic decision, which is one that is consistent with the way the client lived his or her life and the values reflected by that life.

When decisions must be made for infants and others who have never been mentally competent, the best interest standard is used, which requires surrogates to decide based on what would be in the person's best interest. If nurses or other professional care-givers become concerned that the next of kin is not deciding based on the clients' values, wishes, and best interest, or there is disagreement among family members as to what the client would have wanted, a guardian *ad litem* will be appointed by the courts as a proxy decision maker.

Normally, a client's wife would have the authority to make decisions for her incompetent husband. The client's wife in the preceding case appears to be doing her best to act in accordance with her husband's values and wishes, but her judgment raises serious concerns. The nurse must ultimately decide if this constitutes elder neglect. If, in fact, this incident is part of a larger pattern of similar incidents, it should be reported. But if there is no clear evidence of neglect, the question remains: How should decisions be made for this client?

The key to resolving this problem is to attend to the client's relationship to his wife and the significance that relationship holds for both of them. The risks posed by the bad judgment of the client's wife may be mitigated by the benefits of keeping the client at home. Thus, the challenge is to find a way to help maintain the client's relationship to his wife while acting to address the concerns about his safety. In general, the first step is to consider ways to make it possible for him to remain safely at home as long as possible. The nurse could talk with the client's wife to explore creative ways to deal with the difficulties of caring for him and to suggest the options available, such as a home health aide. She could help her develop a plan to deal with emergencies. She could also begin preparing his wife for the time when home health care will no longer be feasible. Because the bad judgment of the care-giver could eventually place the client in such danger that it must be reported, this situation requires close monitoring. Currently, however, home health care agencies are not reimbursed for visits simply to monitor a situation.

> This client is off service for a while, but then she's back again. She has coronary disease, long-standing diabetes, and peripheral vascular disease. She's really confused. She grimaces and then denies she's in pain. She thinks she goes off to the office every day, but she never leaves the house. I personally think she's incompetent. Right now she has a black toe. She was admitted to the hospital two days ago, and the doctor wanted to amputate. But he asked her daughter, and she refused permission. Now she's home again and back on service. I scheduled a visit today, but her daughter met me at the door and told me, "I'll handle my mother." She wouldn't let me in. **What responsibilities do I have when the client's daughter refuses to let me care for my client?**

A nurse's responsibility is to act to ensure that clients receive the care they require. If the nurse is unable to see this client to provide that care herself, her professional responsibility nevertheless requires that she act to protect the client's well-being. She could follow-up with an attempt to reach the client directly, perhaps with a phone call, and try to schedule another visit. She should also report this incident to the appropriate supervisor and the client's physician.

Though the nurse believes the client is incompetent, apparently no formal determination has been made in this case. As often happens, physicians have turned to the adult daughter to make decisions about the client's care. In light of her refusal to give permission for the surgery and her refusal to admit the nurse to see her mother, the daughter's decision-making authority should be questioned. Because she appears to be seriously jeopardizing her mother's well-being, this may constitute elder abuse, which would have to be reported.

WITHHOLDING INFORMATION AND DECEIVING OTHERS

Doctors often leave it to the nurse to explain things. Recently I started caring for a woman with three young children who has just been diagnosed with breast cancer that has metastasized to the lungs. Her physician has scheduled her for a radiation procedure with a gamma knife. I know she is not a candidate because she has multiple tumors in her lungs. I confronted her doctor: "You know she's not a candidate. Why did you schedule this?" He said, "I want to give her hope." **Should I go along with deceiving a client in order to give her hope?**

Cases like this are often referred to as "benevolent deception," that is, deception that is intended to benefit the client. Do the benefits justify this deception? In order to answer this question it is necessary to recognize that truth-telling in client care is important because of the right of self-determination. Individuals cannot make adequate decisions for themselves if they do not have the relevant information, or if the information they have is false or biased.

The client's right of self-determination is recognized in the legal doctrine of informed consent, which requires physicians to disclose to the client: (1) the diagnosis; (2) the prognosis with and without the proposed treatment; and (3) the alternatives to treatment, including risks and benefits of each alternative. There must be disclosure of any information that is *material* to a treatment decision before seeking the client's consent.

Determining whether information is material requires analyzing two components— probability and consequences. Thus, the client needs to be provided with all information that will enable her to take into account the risks of the procedure in relation to the severity of possible injury and the likelihood that the injury will occur. Everyday risks, such as the possibility of surgery-related infection, need not be disclosed.

There are two different standards that courts have used to determine a duty to disclose medical information. The first is the professional or medical community model. Under this standard of disclosure, the doctor is required to disclose only those risks that are consistent with the practice of the local community. The question is whether the physician proceeds as other competent medical professionals would in a similar situation.

The second standard is the reasonable patient standard. This standard asks what an objective reasonable patient would consider to be relevant to the decision to consent or refuse. Doctors may not withhold information because of their own discomfort or because full disclosure might result in the patient's decision to forego treatment. Withholding the truth under such circumstances would constitute negligence, making the doctor liable for damages.

When a physician uses benevolent deception to give a client hope, the nurse's appropriate ethical response is to confront the physician and express concerns about meeting the requirement for informed consent. Truly informed consent requires that clients be provided with honest alternatives, that is, options that are realistically expected to be of some benefit to the client. That has not happened in this case. Because it compromises the possibility of informed consent, this deception is ostensibly wrong.

This case also presents an issue about character. The physician has involved the nurse in his attempts at benevolent deception, without her prior knowledge or consent. This raises the important question whether the nurse should reveal the physician's well-intentioned deception. How can she respond with compassion for the client, but still be honest? It seems clear that nurses should not deceive clients, even in order to give them hope, and they should object to any physicians' attempts to deceive. If asked directly, nurses should not lie to clients, but volunteering information could create a conflict with the physician. The nurse could suggest that the client ask the doctor for more exact information about her condition and prognosis.

This case demonstrates the integral though sometimes unacknowledged role nurses often play in informed consent. Clients expect them to explain what physicians have left unexplained, to clarify and interpret what their physicians have told them, and to answer the questions they may hesitate to ask their physicians. This role is enhanced in home health care because clients see doctors less frequently than when they are hospitalized.

> One of my clients is an elderly woman who broke her collar bone. Her daughter told me that the doctor said her mother also had an aneurysm and won't live long. The mother is nervous and easily upset, so her doctor has decided to tell her nothing about this. Now her daughter is insisting that I promise I won't say anything to the other nurses. She's afraid her mother will find out. **When is it permissible to withhold information from a competent client? Is it ever permissible to withhold information from other health care professionals?**

There are three exceptions to legal rules regarding informed consent and disclosure of information to patients. The first is when the patient is unconscious or otherwise incompetent to make a decision, and the harm from failure to treat is both imminent and outweighs the harm likely to be brought about by the treatment itself. In situations where the patient is unconscious and immediate treatment is required, courts have agreed that physicians can act without informed consent as long as treatment is in accordance with standard emergency practice. Going further, some courts have held that informed consent is implied in all emergency situations.

The second exception, relevant in this case, involves the notion of therapeutic privilege. This concept acknowledges that, at times, disclosure of medical information renders patients incapable of rational decision making, complicates or hinders treatment, or perhaps even poses psychological damage to the patient.

Therapeutic privilege is a controversial exception, and the law is unclear as to its scope. As such, this "privilege" must be carefully circumscribed. Nurses should scrutinize any claims of therapeutic privilege and clarify with physicians the basis for considering information harmful if therapeutic privilege is claimed. The exception is justified only if there are compelling reasons for believing disclosure will harm the client. Otherwise, nurses should advocate for truthful disclosure.

The third exception to the doctrine of informed consent occurs when a competent patient waives the right to receive medical information. A waiver is the voluntary and intentional relinquishment of a known right.

In this case, there do appear to be grounds for withholding the diagnosis based on the daughter's assessment of the emotional and psychological state of the client. Regrettably, the client will then be denied the opportunity to address any "unfinished business" before she dies, which presumably would be important to her. The significance of this should be discussed with her daughter.

Should a nurse withhold this information from other nurses? The answer is an unequivocal "no." A nurse would be guilty of unprofessional conduct if she filed a false report or record in the practice of nursing, or if she failed to furnish appropriate details about a client's nursing needs to other nurses involved in providing continuing nursing services.

I have a young boy, a teenager, with brain cancer. This is hard. His parents know he's dying, but they won't let us address that. They won't even let the chaplain come in to see him. There's always a parent in the room. He's been asking questions, but they always step in and stop the discussion. I think he'd like honest answers, but they won't allow it. **Should children be told the truth?**

Because minors are not allowed to make medical decisions, it may seem that they do not need to be told the truth. After all, the legal basis for requiring truthful disclosure is to promote an informed decision. Yet it does not seem right to lie or withhold the truth, especially from an older child who possesses the decision-making capabilities of an adult.

In fact, psychological studies show that children recognize subtle cues in such cases; they frequently know more about their illness than others expect. Children often have what is referred to as "closed awareness"—they know they are seriously ill, but they do not discuss it openly. Some families prefer to cope with serious illness and impending death in this way.

On the other hand, some would maintain that even young children have the right to know about their illnesses in language suited to their age. Nurses may prefer dealing with minors who are informed about their illnesses; nonetheless, the decision to disclose information is the parents' decision to make. In any case, nurses should not deceive a child, though they are expected to refrain from volunteering information to a young child. They should defer to parents to answer any significant questions children have.

Older children can show remarkable abilities to understand their situation, even when their illness is not treatable. Thus, a stronger case can be made for truthfulness when the client is a teenager, for example, as in the case preceding. Given the fact that he is persistently questioning the nurse and seems to want honest answers, the nurse should advocate for disclosure of information. She may also want to discuss with the parents the advantages of promoting his understanding so that he can openly discuss his concerns and fears, and contribute to the end of life decisions that will be required on his behalf.

There are special legal considerations relating to minors, though the doctrine of informed consent does not apply to them directly. Except in special circumstances minors cannot give valid consent for medical procedures for themselves; parents or guardians must give proxy consent for them. Because parents are presumed to act in the best interest of their children, courts endow them with broad decision making authority. The government or courts can restrict parents' rights only if they have a compelling interest, such as the preservation of life and prevention of suicide, safeguarding against physical or emotional abuse or neglect, the protection of innocent third parties, or maintenance of the integrity of the medical profession. Otherwise, parents have the right to raise their children as they see fit.

There are several circumstances, however, in which minors are allowed to consent for themselves. For purely pragmatic reasons, most states allow minors to give their own consent for conditions that pose risks to public health and that might go untreated if the minor had to get parental consent. These include treatment for substance abuse and venereal disease. Some minors have the legal status of emancipated minors, meaning that they have all the rights and responsibilities of adults. This status is conferred if they are in the armed forces, or married, or if they have in court proven economic independence from their parents.

In addition, some states recognize certain individuals as mature minors for the purpose of consenting to their own treatment. This usually follows the recommendation of a physician who testifies that they can demonstrate an understanding of the nature and consequences of treatment or refusal and can exercise the judgment of an adult.

A less formal substitute for informed consent is the requirement of informed assent. Federal regulations require that children over the age of seven be informed about their treatment in age appropriate language and be asked for their assent. Even without assent, beneficial treatment can be provided if parents consent. Only in nontherapeutic research does the child's refusal serve as a veto to participation.

ETHICAL CRITERIA

- The competent client has a right to make free, deliberate, and informed decisions.
- The client has a right to truthful information.

PRACTICAL STRATEGIES

When the client lives alone:

1. Educate the client about any risks involved.
2. Determine alternatives to risky situations.
3. Act to make the environment safer.

When clients are unrealistic:

1. Educate clients about the nature and risks of their situation.
2. Ask permission to raise the issue with the family caregiver.

When clients live dangerously:

1. Ensure that the client is competent and that decisions are fully informed.
2. Explain risks and alternatives.
3. Act to diminish the risks.
4. Attempt to persuade the client to avoid risks.
5. Intervene when the risks involve others.

When clients' families create risks:

1. Educate clients and family members about the risks.
2. Ask the client's permission to raise the issue with others.
3. Suggest actions to diminish the risks.
4. Report to your supervisor when the risk seems unacceptable.

When clients are incompetent:

1. Assure that there is a competent caregiver.
2. Advocate for decisions that agree with the client's known wishes and values.
3. Contact supervisors and outside agencies when caregivers abuse or neglect the client.

When physicians withhold information:

1. Discuss the reasons for withholding information with the physician.
2. Advocate for truthful disclosure.
3. Encourage the client to ask questions.

When families withhold information:

1. Explore what the client wants to know through questioning.
2. Answer the client's questions honestly.
3. Educate the family about the client's right to truthful information.

When therapeutic privilege is cited as a reason for withholding information:

1. Discuss with the physician the reasons the information is considered harmful.
2. Advocate for disclosure of as much truthful information as possible.
3. Communicate truthfully with all members of the health care team.

When parents withhold information from a minor:

1. Advocate for truthful disclosure of information appropriate to minor's maturity.
2. Educate parents about the costs and benefits of nondisclosure.

Chapter 3

THE ROLE OF THE FAMILY

You need to have families involved in home health care, but it doesn't always work out well. Right now I am caring for a man who had a devastating stroke. His son moved him into his house to care for him. My client complained to me that his son is not bathing him often enough or feeding him regularly. Then he started to cry and said he didn't want to do anything to upset his son. He needs nursing care, but now his son wants to stop the home health care visits. **Should his son be the one to make these decisions?**

General Issues

- **What is the role of the family in decision making?**
- **What is the nurse's responsibility when families jeopardize the client's well-being?**
- **What should nurses do when family disagreements affect the client's care?**
- **What are the limits of obligations to caregivers?**

INTRODUCTION

When illness or injury strikes, the decisions clients make and the care they receive can be profoundly influenced by their families. This influence is limited in some ways if clients are hospitalized. Issues about families and their proper role in decisions can arise in that setting, but families cannot ordinarily deny the hospitalized client's right to decide nor interfere directly with the care the client receives. Clients are not as isolated from their families' influence in the home setting where families usually have a substantial role in providing care.

26

Exemplary family caregivers are devoted, competent, and responsible. However, a family's response to illness and the responsibilities of caring for someone who is ill or dying can vary greatly. In truth, some family caregivers may actually be psychologically and emotionally incapable of providing the intimate, personal care required. Families are also at times intolerant of the changes that illness can produce. Moreover, all the unresolved conflicts inherent in family relationships can be exacerbated by the stress of illness. Adult children, for example, may harbor resentments that complicate their involvement in caring for their parents. Clients, too, respond in different ways to their illnesses. Some find it particularly difficult to accept help from their families, while others demand their unstinting attention and care. Home health care nurses practice in a setting where concerns about the role of the family are the source of daunting issues about nurses' responsibilities.

THE FAMILY'S ROLE IN DECISION MAKING

One of my clients is a woman who has no mobility from the waist down. She can't get out of bed to her wheelchair. Three weeks ago she was diagnosed with a very serious decubitus. I see her five days a week for the dressing changes she needs for the bed sores. Her husband washes her and changes the dressing in the morning before he goes to work and again when he gets home. He doesn't get her out of bed, though. She's in bed all day; what she needs is to be up for an hour, back in bed an hour, then up again. There are three adult children living nearby, but they have not helped at all. He's burning out. He can't keep her at home like she wants and continue to work at the job he has. **What role should I encourage a family to take when decisions like this have to be made?**

Because family caregivers often have a critical role in home health care, clients' decisions about care will have a clear impact on them. The integral role of the family raises issues about how these decisions should be made and whether families should be involved. Even for competent clients who are capable of making decisions for themselves, there are different ways in which decision making can be conceptualized.

a. *Individualistic decision making.* The moral and legal requirements for informed consent appear to assume that clients' decisions are purely unilateral and individual. When a decision is necessary, clients think through the issues independently and reach a decision. Clients are free to choose among different treatments, or to refuse any and all treatment, informed by medical information and their own set of values.

There is a problem with this model. Though some decisions seem to have implications only for a client, most decisions will have an impact on others, especially in the home health care setting. For example, a client's decision to reject transfer to a rehabilitation center or nursing home means, in effect, that someone must be willing and able to continue to care for the client at home. In some cases this kind of decision would require a family member who is ill or already overwhelmed to accept this responsibility. Of course, the right to choose obviously cannot include the right to make impossible demands on others. Moreover, because all individuals are involved in relationships, a totally individualistic model of decision making does not reflect the reality of people's lives.

b. *Collaborative decision making.* In collaborative decision making, clients retain their central role in making final decisions for themselves but reach their decisions after consultation with their families. This process is particularly useful when clients are unsure about their own wishes. Family members are asked to share their own views about what it would be best for the client to do and to contribute ideas that could aid the client in reaching a decision. At the end of the process the client makes a decision based on the discussion.

Consider, for example, an older man who must decide whether to continue to live with his son or accept placement in a nursing home. He knows his son will not be able to provide the same level of care that he would receive in an institution where professional staff are present. Consequently, he knows he is risking his health to some extent if he remains at home. If he is not sure what to do, he could consult with his son and they could discuss the possibilities together. Gradually, through sharing their ideas, they should be able to clarify his options and his wishes. They may determine that he really wants to stay with his son, despite the limitations that involves. They could then conclude that it is a reasonable choice for him. Although it remains his decision, they have come to the decision together.

On this model, clients see themselves not as isolated individuals, but as members of a family that operates as a community. They recognize family relationships as important to their thinking. The limitation of this model is that it works only when there are good relationships among those involved.

c. *Compromise decision making.* On this model, competent clients who have clear ideas about what they want are willing to shape their decisions in response to the wishes of others. Individuals and family members begin this process by sharing their ideas of what they each want to happen. Through negotiation and compromise, each is persuaded to yield in some way. The client is able to make a decision that is as close to his or her original wish as is practically feasible, but that still responds to the concerns of others.

Compromise decision making could be utilized in the preceding case. Though the client wants to remain at home, her husband is not able to provide care during the day unless he takes time off from work. Their adult children have not yet been involved in caring for their mother. The client, her husband, and children might compromise in the following way. The husband and children could agree to share the daily task of caring for the client, each providing a few hours of care one day a week, with a promise to rethink this if the arrangement imposes too great a burden on any of them. The clients' children thus accept some responsibility for their mother's care, and her husband agrees to take more time off from work than he would like. The advantage of this kind of decision making is that it recognizes the client as the final decision maker, but allows for input from others and seeks a solution that works for everyone. The disadvantage is that in some cases the individuals may be so far apart or so adamant in their original positions that compromise is impossible.

When decisions must be made, nurses should help families understand that, from both a moral and legal perspective, the client is the final decision maker. Nevertheless, clients should be encouraged to weigh the impact their individual decisions will have on others. Nurses should also encourage clients and families to recognize that their relationships are an important factor to consider when addressing issues about decisions.

> I have a really difficult case right now, a young client who is dying from colon cancer. Her husband hardly leaves her side. He complains she's sleeping all the time, and he wants to spend time with her. He doesn't want us stepping up her morphine even though she's in pain. **Should he have the right to decide what medications she receives?**

Though this client is not now competent to decide for herself, any decisions that are made on her behalf should respect her prior expressions of wishes concerning treatment in such circumstances. In past conversations or past experiences with illness, did she ever express her feelings about receiving large amounts of pain medication, even if it would sedate her to the point of unconsciousness? If any information about her wishes is available, then it is possible to use the standard of substituted judgment to make the decision she would make if she could. Without any information concerning a client's wishes, treatment decisions should be made on the basis of the best interest standard. Calculating a client's best interest can require attention to particular circumstances and the effect of any decision on relationships, as well as addressing the client's need for relief from pain. Without convincing information that additional time with her husband is more important to the client's best interest than pain relief, the husband's decision cannot be justified.

It is possible that he does not realize how close to death she is and how much pain she is experiencing. In such circumstances nurses should focus on educating the caregiver about the reality of the situation and attempt to motivate actions based on compassion for the client. This might lead to a satisfactory resolution.

Under the best of circumstances the client and her husband would have discussed the choices that need to be made for her and could have used compromise decision making to reach mutually agreeable conclusions about her care at the end of life. If that process had resulted in her decision to stay conscious for as long as possible, her husband's actions would be reasonable. Otherwise, the husband's insistence that his wife be conscious violates her presumed best interest and should be resisted. If necessary, the nurse could contact her supervisor at the agency with any concerns she has about this family member's decisions concerning medications. Discussions with the agency's ethics advisory committee, if it has one, would also be helpful.

Ethics committees began to develop in hospitals in the 1970s. They were charged with overseeing decisions concerning matters of life and death where there was likely to be a conflict in values. Since then, ethics committees have been involved in client and community education, retrospective and prospective case review and consultation, and, in some cases, policy development. The membership of ethics committees varies, but often these committees include physicians, nurses, lawyers, philosophers, clergy, and community representatives. Most ethics committees have engaged in extensive discussions of treatment decisions regarding the seriously ill, what constitutes futile treatment, and when do not resuscitate orders are justified. More recent debates focus on responsibilities to indigent clients and what to do with the growing number of psychiatric patients for whom there are no transfer facilities available.

In addition to wrestling with these issues, home health care ethics committees face dilemmas uniquely related to the setting. These involve not only the context of the practice, but the reliance on a team of formal and informal caregivers, challenges related to safety in an environment that is difficult to regulate, and the complexities of reimbursement in an era of managed care.

WHEN FAMILIES JEOPARDIZE THE CLIENT'S WELLBEING

I have a client whose wife second guesses the doctors. She tries to control everything that happens. She prepours his medications. I found out she had doubled up on the Lasix, which affects potassium levels. She said, "Don't worry, I have potassium pills I'm giving him, too." I have tried to explain that her interference with his medications may be harmful, but she says she knows him better than we do. I know she is doing what she thinks is best for him, still it's dangerous for her to play doctor like this. **How can I guarantee that the client gets the care he needs?**

Troubling issues about the actions of family caregivers can arise even when families are well meaning and believe they are doing what is best for the client. Families many times feel they know what a client needs better than the doctors do. When this occurs, it is important for nurses to determine why a caregiver believes a dosage should be adjusted or omitted. The client's wife may have noticed a change that led her to conclude that the medications should be increased. If so, she should bring those changes to the attention of the nurse so that the nurse can assess the need for a change in medication or dosage and contact the physician if necessary. Because his wife appears to be sincerely concerned about the client's well-being, effective teaching about the dangers of adjusting his medications in this way should help to resolve this problem.

I can't believe some families. One of my clients is very wealthy. He came on the service for wound care. Medicare pays for that. He also has round-the-clock nursing care he's paying for, but his nephew has power of attorney over his financial affairs. After the first bill arrived and he saw how much it cost, his nephew decided his uncle just needs the daytime nurse covered by Medicare. Now he has his friends coming in to care for his uncle. He said he's afraid his uncle's funds will run out. The funds will never run out! I know the uncle won't say anything because he doesn't want to end up in a nursing home. **Is this any of my business? Should I keep my concerns to myself?**

Home health care nurses have the responsibility of determining when the behavior of families justifies intervening on behalf of clients. In this case, the client has the right to reduce or eliminate nursing services as long as he is competent and fully aware of his medical condition. Here, however, it is not clear that the client has freely agreed to this, because he needs his nephew's cooperation to be able to remain in his own home. Does this amount to coercion? That's a hard call to make. The situation of being ill is itself coercive because the choices people can make are so limited. There is also an unspoken threat from the nephew that the client would have to go to a nursing home if he wants to continue with round-the-clock nursing care. This increases the possibility that his acceptance of this change is not fully voluntary. The nurse can support the uncle's right to self-determination by reminding the nephew that the client should make these decisions. She should also talk to the client about his wishes. It is possible that the client is willing to accept less nursing care and comfort in exchange for being able to remain in his own home. If that is the case, the nurse should ensure that he understands the consequences of his decision. If he freely decides to go along with his nephew's dictum, then that is his choice.

The possibility of elder abuse and neglect must also be considered in cases like this. Elder abuse and neglect includes both physical and emotional harm, comprised of physical assault, verbal and sexual abuse, isolation, confinement, and financial exploitation. Such crimes against elders, like crimes against children, are deemed worthy of special consideration because the victims are considered more vulnerable and have a greater degree of dependence. Therefore, they warrant additional protection through the coercive power of the law. The problem is that after the nurses have been discharged, there may be no one in a position to monitor the client's condition.

WHEN FAMILY DISAGREEMENTS AFFECT
THE CLIENT'S CARE

Sometimes family conflicts sabotage the plan of care. One of my clients is a widower who has lived alone for years. His daughter lived out of state. When he got sick, she moved back home. He doesn't want any further treatment, but his daughter won't accept that. She calls him a "coward" and a "quitter" for not fighting. He told me not to do anything about it, just to "let his daughter be." **Should I try to get her to accept her father's decision or let them work it out?**

As an advocate for the client's right to self-determination, nurses should promote actions in accord with the client's decisions. In this instance, the client has decided to forego further treatment, a decision that should be respected. However, his daughter apparently does not share the same perspective on his illness and the plan of care. The question is whether nurses should get involved in this family matter, beyond clarifying with the daughter the client's right to make these decisions. Historically, nurses have considered families to be an important part of their care, a focus that is quite naturally enhanced when they practice in the home health care setting.

The key to this situation lies in recognizing that the client is an individual involved in relationships, rather than an isolated individual. The consequences for the client's relationships should be considered when determining whether to do more than simply support the client's right to self-determination. Clearly, the client would benefit from his daughter's acceptance of his decisions about treatment and the improved relationship that would result. To that end, the nurse could, with the client's permission, discuss with the daughter the reality of the situation and attempt to lead her to accept and support her father's decision. However, if the client does not agree to allow this discussion, the nurse should leave it to them to work out on their own. It is important to note that nurses cannot discuss the client's health without permission, even with family members, because of a client's right to confidentiality.

Some families really get in the way. I have a client with esophageal cancer. He says the care that he is getting is fine, but his daughter hates us. She makes all the decisions. The sicker he gets, the harder it is to deal with her. None of the nurses want to go there. When I got there yesterday, she met me at the door and shouted, "He's dying. What the hell are you going to do about it?" I want out, but I think the agency will drop him if one more nurse quits this case. **What should I do?**

Despite the best efforts of nurses, conflicts may arise between nurses and families that can affect a client's health. The tension and unhappiness in this household adds to the client's stress and could diminish his ability to face his prognosis. When a family's behavior is harming a client in this way, a nurse has the obligation to act on behalf of the client. She should attempt to discuss this with the client's daughter and to explain the harm this behavior causes. However, the nurse's own ability to help is limited, given the daughter's hostility to her. One course of action would be to recommend counseling to help the daughter control her feelings of hostility, because her expression of anger is a recognized stage of the grieving process. A social worker could help her understand the impact on her father and help her develop appropriate coping skills.

Finally, no one is expected to work under abusive conditions. Nurses can justifiably quit a case, assuming that they follow the appropriate steps in accordance with agency policy and state law. Because several nurses have already quit the case, the agency is unlikely to want to continue to keep this client on service. Nonetheless, this nurse does not have a special obligation to tolerate hostility and to continue caring for the client. If she decides to continue on this case, her actions are supererogatory, that is, above and beyond what is morally required.

One of my clients wants so much to please her family, she is not able to communicate honestly when they are there. She's declining but the family is in denial. They are intense, very protective. They hover around her and prevent her from talking to me. With me, she's reviewing her life. I don't think the family wants to let her do that. **How can I help the client when her family won't allow it?**

Silent, unacknowledged conflicts between clients and families are the source of real quandaries when nurses are prevented from acting in the client's best interests. Resolving such quandaries requires attention to the client's wishes and the value the client places on family relationships.

Clients sometimes make decisions that benefit their families, but at the same time harm their own interests. For example, some clients want their families to be able to deny what is happening when they are seriously ill, because they think this makes it easier for the family. As a consequence, they relinquish any opportunity to discuss with their families matters that are important to them when they are dying.

Though this client could possibly benefit if the family were not in denial about the reality of her situation, she should be the one to determine whether the nurse discusses this matter with anyone in the family. The nurse could offer to talk with the family for her, with her permission, or offer to be present to help her broach the subject with them herself. This would free them to talk to each other about any important issues, if they wish to do so.

But if the client wishes to allow the family to deny how sick she is, then the nurse should respect that wish. Her only option then is to attempt to secure private time for the client to have the opportunity to ask her questions and express her feelings. This must be done in a way that does not upset the client's family or interfere with the client's relationship with her family.

> I really don't understand families who can't put aside their differences when someone is dying. It is tough when they don't get along. I have a Lupus client who is dying. She wants to see her mother but her husband refuses to allow it. He's never forgiven her mother for something that happened years ago. I want to help her but I don't want to get in the middle of a family feud. **How far does my responsibility to my client extend?**

A nurse could justifiably consider this concern to lie outside her professional duty to provide skilled nursing care. As an advocate for her client, though, she may have a responsibility to address a situation that will cause considerable distress for her.

One way to approach this issue would be to reflect on the behavior that would best satisfy her professional ideals as a nurse. An important objective is to become a caring nurse who acts to ease the suffering of her clients. For this client, easing her suffering means seeking a way to help her see her mother. The nurse should obviously only take action with the client's permission, though. First, she could talk with the client's husband to impress on him the gravity of the situation and how important it is for the client to see her mother before she dies. Second, if the client requests it, she could consider contacting the client's mother herself. Whatever action she does take, she must weigh carefully the possible consequences for the client's relationship to her husband.

THE LIMITS OF OBLIGATIONS TO CAREGIVERS

Sometimes we go into cases and it turns out that the caregiver needs more help than the person we're assigned to. I have an Alzheimer's patient. Whenever his wife is in the room, he becomes difficult. She is in her eighties, but when he starts acting up she needs to leave the house. She'll drive around for hours at a time. Her children want to put him in a nursing home. She told me she can't do that. "I took a vow." She can't cope, but she refuses to admit it. **How do I balance my responsibilities to the caregiver and to the client?**

Though nurses are primarily client advocates, home health care nurses do have an obligation to act on behalf of caregivers if their health or safety is endangered. Indeed, everyone has a moral obligation to prevent harm to others when it is possible to do so without substantial sacrifice or great difficulty. Part of the nurse's responsibility in this case, then, is to discuss frankly with the client's wife the risk to her own well-being if the client remains at home. Nevertheless, she may prefer to take that risk rather than place her husband in a nursing home. If that is the case, the nurse could seek additional services such as respite care to help her cope with the burden of caring for her husband. For a moral perspective, nurses do have a responsibility to respond to these concerns about a caregiver.

This case raises questions about client safety and well-being, as well. If the limitations of the caregiver pose a risk of harm to the client, then the nurse has an obligation to take the appropriate action to protect him.

The very presence of the family or other caregivers, which is the strength of home health care, raises ethical issues that nurses must resolve. Although families are often strong allies of health care professionals, they can present obstacles to good nursing care. Nurses must achieve a delicate balance between respecting caregivers for the important role they play and advocating for clients who are very dependent on the abilities and good will of others.

ETHICAL CRITERIA

- Competent clients have the right to make their own decisions.
- Competent clients may voluntarily relinquish that right to someone else.

PRACTICAL STRATEGIES

When the client's decisions significantly affect the family:

1. Encourage the client to recognize how decisions affect the family.
2. Promote collaborative or compromise decision making.

When the family interferes with the plan of care:

1. Educate the family about the reasons for the prescribed plan of care.
2. Advocate for the client's best interest.
3. Acknowledge and support the family's efforts to care for the client.

When the family's motives and decisions raise concerns:

1. Ask a competent client's permission before raising these issues with the family.
2. Ensure the client's safety needs and best interests are served.
3. Contact the appropriate authorities when abuse and neglect are suspected.
4. Provide information on resources and support services for families.
5. Encourage the family to respect a competent client's wishes.

When the family caregiver cannot cope:

1. Inform the caregiver about alternatives and support services.
2. Take appropriate action if the caregiver's limitations pose a risk of harm to the client.

Chapter 4

SAFEGUARDING SECRETS, PROTECTING PRIVACY

One of my HIV patients is a forty-two-year-old male. He is so dysfunctional that he is not able to work. His HIV medications are paid for by a state subsidized AIDS program, which doesn't cover the antidepressants or pain medications he needs. He refuses to let me contact his parents for help. They don't know he is HIV-positive. **Should I talk to them anyway so he gets his medications?**

General Issues

- **Who should have access to information about clients?**
- **When is a nurse justified in breaching confidentiality?**
- **How far should nurses go to protect their clients' privacy?**
- **Does a nurse have a responsibility to protect family privacy?**

INTRODUCTION

Families are usually in a position to know a great deal about the health of clients when they are cared for at home. Caregivers arrive, medical supplies are delivered, nursing schedules change, all under the watchful eyes of clients' families. Even the neighbors might know more than clients want them to know about their health under these circumstances.

What they do not know, families, and sometimes neighbors, expect nurses to reveal if they ask. Nurses are, after all, working in the client's home, which families commonly regard as their own domain. Families may also have an opportunity to gain access to confidential medical information from any medical record or travel chart that is kept in the home. This is a special concern when sensitive personal matters are documented. Given the access families usually have to information about home health care clients, and their presumption that nurses should provide whatever further medical information they seek, maintaining confidentiality is more difficult than it is when clients are hospitalized.

Protecting the privacy of home health care clients is also challenging. Nurses have access to more personal information about clients and their families when they are cared for in their own homes than they would generally be in a position to have in a hospital setting. They know more about their clients' lifestyles and personal habits, their financial circumstances, family relationships, and family "secrets." Any immoral or illegal activities may be difficult for clients and families to conceal from nurses, simply because nurses are present in the home. Nurses' access to private information and family secrets raises the issue of what to document and what secrets to keep.

ACCESS TO INFORMATION ABOUT CLIENTS

When I go to the HIV clinic, they're all my patients. They say "hello," so everyone else knows they have AIDS. They couldn't care less about confidentiality. They all know each other, so they ask: "How's so-and-so doing?" **Can I tell them anything?**

Though it may seem harmless to answer that question about how a client is doing, it would be a violation of confidentiality. From a legal point of view, confidentiality is protected by privileged communication statutes. The nurse-patient relationship, like the physician-patient relationship, is a confidential one. This means that nurses must refrain from discussing patients with third parties, regardless of their benign intentions. A nurse who breaches this confidence commits a tort, which is a violation of an individual's legal rights. Depending on the jurisdiction in which the complaint is filed and the circumstances involved, a nurse could be charged with breach of confidence, breach of contract, or invasion of privacy for revealing confidential medical information, including the very fact that an individual is her patient.

When clients are terminal, they don't want their families to know how close to death they are. They want them to enjoy life, they don't want them to be depressed. A client with bowel cancer that had metastacized told me: "I know I'm dying, but I don't want them to know." He wants to pretend that he is getting better. I think his family should know he's dying. **Should I tell his family the truth?**

Based on their right to self-determination, competent clients have the moral right to determine what medical information about them is confidential, to decide who, if anyone, is to have access to details about their health, and to control the extent of any individual's access to that information. This includes deciding which family members, if any, are informed about the client's medical condition. If they wish, clients can designate someone other than a family member, such as a life partner or a close friend, as a person who should have access to all client information. Families do not generally have the right to choose what information they will have or who should be told the client's diagnosis or prognosis. Clients can indeed refuse permission for any such discussions with their families.

In order to ensure that the client's rights are protected, nurses could ask specific questions in their initial assessment to determine what the client wishes to keep confidential and who the client wishes to have access to medical information. Nurses should also discuss with the client the issue of maintaining the confidentiality of any medical record that remains in the home and their concerns about protecting the client's privacy.

In this case, the nurse cannot reveal the client's terminal prognosis without his permission. However, given that the client, himself, would presumably benefit if his family knew he was dying, the nurse should encourage him to reconsider this. The family, too, might benefit from the opportunity to prepare for his impending death. Though the nurse cannot reveal the prognosis or any confidential information, she nevertheless should not deceive the family herself by providing false information. She could suggest that family members discuss any concerns they have with the client, if they press her for answers to their questions.

BREACHING CONFIDENTIALITY

Recently, a female client fell and broke her hip. We came on service for pain management. Her daughter took her in, but because she works, the client is home alone. She almost fell again this week. I'm concerned that she is not safe by herself, but she doesn't want me to discuss this with her daughter. She said she doesn't want to upset her. **Should I tell her daughter what happened?**

The client would ordinarily have the right to keep this information from her daughter. However, if her safety is at risk, a breach of confidentiality may be justified. From a legal perspective, the only exceptions to the requirement to maintain the confidentiality of medical information are in cases where disclosure is required or authorized by the law. The patient's right to confidentiality is not absolute and may be overridden by the state's duty to protect public health and maintain the integrity of the medical profession. Legally required disclosures of otherwise confidential information fall into three categories: (1) disclosures required by subpoena; (2) those required by statute to protect public health and welfare such as mandates to report births and deaths, communicable diseases, victims of violent assault, or child abuse and neglect; and (3) disclosure necessary to protect the patient or innocent third party from serious and imminent harm.

Although the courts have affirmed the right to disclose confidential medical information in these sets of circumstances, four limitations regulating the release of confidential information have been outlined. Confidential information must be disclosed in good faith and reasonable care should be given to guarantee that it is accurate, reported fairly, limited to what is necessary for the sake of protection, and given only to the people who need it for the purpose of protection.

In deciding cases based on breaches of confidentiality, the courts consider whether the disclosure was malicious or made in good faith. The latter mistake usually involves paying compensatory damages alone, but breaches of confidentiality deemed malicious could result in the revocation of one's license, being forced to pay punitive damages, and in some states criminal prosecution. Health care providers who breach patient confidentiality are at risk of liability for damages related to invasion of privacy, malpractice, intentional infliction of emotional distress, breach of applicable state confidentiality statutes, and breach of contract.

In situations where the question is whether to reveal confidential information for the benefit of the client, the best solution is to persuade clients to reveal the information themselves. Although the client has thus far refused to do this, it is important to explore her reasons for attempting to conceal her injury and deceive her daughter about the risks of staying home alone. She may be afraid of her daughter's reaction when she learns she has nearly fallen again or worried that she will no longer be able to live with her daughter. Whether or not the nurse decides that this situation justifies breaching her client's confidentiality, she should be sensitive to the consequences her actions will have for the client's relationship to her daughter and attempt to minimize any adverse results.

> I have one client, a thirty-two-year-old physician with AIDS, who has moved back home so his parents can take care of him. He refuses to tell them he has AIDS. He doesn't want them to know. He has decided to tell them he has hepatitis because the precautions are the same. He has multiple opportunistic infections and nosebleeds all the time now. **Don't they have a right to know they're dealing with AIDS?**

Here, the client is attempting to keep a potentially explosive secret and to protect his family at the same time. Because both hepatitis and AIDS require universal precautions, his parents will be advised to take the same precautionary measures they would for dealing with AIDS. Of course, he assumes that they will meticulously follow these precautions and avoid exposure to HIV. Given that, should his nurse reveal that he has AIDS?

Courts have permitted medical disclosure to third parties when this disclosure is in their "substantial and valid" interest, though different jurisdictions have come to a variety of conclusions regarding the duty health care professionals have to protect third parties from HIV transmission. For example, the Alaska Supreme Court found that a doctor could reveal his patient's HIV status to the patient's wife, against the patient's wishes, without incurring liability. Other jurisdictions have prohibited the disclosure of such information. Though not uniform, current case law reflects the position that where a health care provider knows or should know that the patient's HIV status poses a serious risk to identifiable third parties, there is a duty to warn these third parties.

Risk to others is an important exception to the legal duty to maintain confidentiality, but the risk must be serious, imminent, and likely to be incurred to justify a breach in confidentiality. There may be no basis for revealing the AIDS diagnosis in this case, because the family has been instructed to follow universal precautions.

Any decision to breach confidentiality in cases like this should weigh the effect on the relationship the client has to his parents. Disclosure of the AIDS diagnosis, and thereby the revelation that their son has deceived them about something this important, would influence this family relationship in a considerable and perhaps unpredictable way, possibly with significant consequences for the client. If a nurse or physician decides to reveal this kind of information, a client first should be given the opportunity to disclose the diagnosis himself, with the clear understanding that confidentiality will be breached if it is necessary to protect his family.

The agency ethics committee could be a good sounding board to discuss this case. It would be helpful to hear how others would weigh the costs and benefits of maintaining confidentiality or, alternatively, revealing the diagnosis against the client's wishes. Although ethics committees typically do not make binding decisions, open discussion can clarify the issues and help an individual nurse determine what other nurses consider acceptable resolutions to this dilemma.

> There are a lot of language barriers. I have a new client, an Hispanic man who is a recent immigrant from the Dominican Republic. He has to learn to give himself insulin injections. When I went to his house I found out that neither he nor his wife can understand English. She got the neighbor to translate. All of a sudden the family kneeled down and started praying! I have no idea what the neighbor was saying. **How can I make sure that the client gets correct information and still protect his confidentiality?**

When nurses and clients do not speak the same language, the ethical and legal requirement to disclose information may compel nurses to use translators. This, in turn, sometimes raises issues about confidentiality, as well as issues about truthful and full disclosure of the information required for consent. The rights of clients can best be protected if a professional interpreter is available to accompany the nurse to a client's home. However, coordinating schedules with interpreters and finding appropriate materials in the client's language can be difficult. The result is that nurses could arrive at a home without the ideal resources to address the needs of the client. Sometimes, as in this case, the language problems are not fully apparent until the initial home visit.

In the absence of a professional interpreter, how can nurses meet the requirements to inform clients and protect client confidentiality?

How can they teach clients what they need to know in order to care for themselves? It seems natural to turn to family members, even children, who speak English to provide the necessary translations. Yet, this solution could violate confidentiality and may compromise informed consent. Family members often are unreliable translators, for they sometimes downplay bad news or are unable to accurately communicate medical information.

Clients relinquish some of their privacy, too, when a family member or neighbors are used as translators. What is most troubling is that they forfeit the opportunity to keep information confidential prior to knowing what will be revealed. This is particularly problematic when children are used to translate. Because it is the client's right to decide whether medical information should be revealed to someone else, the nurse in this case should warn the client that information will be disclosed that he may not want others to know. She could then make it clear that the client can stop the discussion at any point if he should decide that he no longer wishes the details of his medical condition revealed in this way, and they can resume their discussion when a professional interpreter is available. That may be inconvenient, but such steps should be taken if necessary to avoid revealing medical information the client wants to keep confidential.

CONFIDENTIAL INFORMATION AND SUICIDE

I'm very upset about one of my clients, a young man who had testicular cancer. He was living with his parents. He sent me e-mail almost every day. Sometimes he just had questions about his health, but other times he shared very personal stuff. We talked a lot about death. About a month ago I suspected that he was considering suicide, so I had a social worker talk to him. After that he seemed less anxious. He died last Friday. The next day I found a suicide note in my e-mail from him. I know no one suspects this. **Should I tell anyone what I know?**

Because the client in this case did not leave a suicide note for his family to find, it seems reasonable to conclude that he did not want them to know the truth. He was probably concerned about the effect on his parents if they learned he committed suicide. Perhaps he wished to spare them the religious, social, and financial consequences that could follow. Though he did reveal his suicide to his nurse, he apparently expected her to keep his secret.

Ethically, the nurse has the obligation to maintain confidentiality. In addition, because of the stigma associated with suicide, the nurse may feel that she should keep her client's secret. In the absence of any overt medical evidence indicating suicide, it would be easy for her to do so. From a legal perspective, however, there is an obligation to produce evidence of the mode of death of the individual. Failure to do so could be regarded as an obstruction of justice. Here is a situation where law and morality seem to conflict. The nurse is legally bound to report the suicide to the authorities, but she is bound by confidentiality to avoid disclosing directly to the family what her client wanted to be kept a secret. She will probably be unable to prevent the family from finding out if she does reveal what she knows. There is no easy resolution to the dilemma in this situation.

> I have a client who has end-stage cirrhosis. He lives with his son. Yesterday he said, "I think I'll shoot myself." He is not crazy, he has just decided that he's had enough. I know he hasn't told anyone else this. I said to his son, "He's dying. You don't know what he might do." **Should I say anything else?**

Another legal exception to the duty to maintain confidentiality exists when clients threaten suicide. Both legally and professionally, nurses are required to report to the physician a client's threats of suicide. The physician must then make a decision regarding detention and civil commitment based on the likelihood of imminent harm to self. Physicians are responsible for knowing and abiding by the procedures governing civil commitment, but it is unlikely that this client would be considered mentally ill and subject to involuntary commitment for his remarks.

Many medical professionals, nurses and others, are convinced that it is possible for a client to make a rational decision that the burdens of continued existence outweigh the benefits. Others take the position that anyone who threatens or attempts suicide is necessarily depressed or mentally incompetent, thus denying the possibility of a rational suicide. On this view, paternalistic intervention would always be warranted. On the whole, contemporary law reflects the position that the duty to prevent suicide generally overrides a client's right to make such a decision, even if it is considered rational. Apart from her legal obligation to report this to his physician, is there anything else that the nurse should do or say? How she responds is a reflection of her character. If she ignores his comment about shooting himself, she neglects her moral and professional obligation to safeguard her client's well-being. She should thus respond in whatever way she can to help him. It is primarily important to address any depression, frustration, or pain that is causing his dissatisfaction with his life under these conditions. She could recommend that he talk to a social worker about his concerns. Finally, the nurse should discuss with the client the effect his suicide would have on his family. Perhaps the client has not thought carefully about these consequences. Under the circumstances, although it would be a breach of confidentiality to say anything else to his son, it may be justified on the grounds that it is necessary to protect the client.

PROTECTING A CLIENT'S PRIVACY

One of my clients is a Cambodian man who is on service for wound care and dressing changes. There are always a lot of people there when I arrive; they feel they need to be there. It's a cultural thing. The patient is very uncomfortable with this but he won't say anything to them. He really has no privacy at all. **Should I do something to protect his privacy when he allows them to stay?**

Based on the right to self-determination, competent clients have the right to determine who have should have access to their private sphere. Therefore, clients should be afforded the opportunity to decide who has access to the most personal information about them and access to their bodies to the extent that it is possible. Under ordinary circumstances, nurses should accept clients' decisions concerning who should be present when caring for them.

The idea that an individual should be afforded privacy for treatment is often an alien idea in cultures that have strong social communities. In these communities, an individual is expected to welcome the constant presence of others throughout an illness and recuperation. The expectations engendered by these cultural practices can complicate a nurse's attempts to preserve the privacy of home health care clients.

The apparent discomfort of the client in this case implies that he may wish more privacy than the practices of his cultural group permit. This justifies the nurse's efforts to enhance his privacy in any way that she can. She should provide the client an opportunity to express his thoughts about this and make it clear that the decision to allow any one else to be there is his decision alone. These efforts must be undertaken with sensitivity to the significance of the expectations and practices of his culture.

> I'm taking care of a teenager who was in a bad car accident. She may not be able to walk normally again. I can't talk with her about it because one of her parents is always there. They never leave us alone. I think she needs some time to talk about her injury and her fears, but they won't allow her to do that. **Should I ask them to leave us alone?**

Though this teenager is not an adult, she is old enough to deserve some privacy when she receives nursing care. More important, she should be able to discuss her prognosis and concerns and assent to any decisions made about her care. Her parents are effectively preventing her involvement in those matters by their presence. They are in fact interfering with the nurse-client relationship by refusing to allow their daughter to have any private time with the nurse. The nurse should urge the parents to respect their daughter's privacy, and she should support the daughter's involvement in medical decisions. The nurse can offer to contact a social worker who can help the family address these issues.

The question of privacy for young teens depends in part on how mature they are. Nurses can offer to answer questions, which allows them to gauge whether the teen would welcome an opportunity to talk privately. Parents may need to be educated about the issue of privacy and the psychological needs of a young teen who faces illness, injury or disability.

PROTECTING FAMILY PRIVACY

> I'm very careful about what I document. I'm an invited guest in a client's home. It is not a public place. I have one situation where the client's son is bizarre. He's taking good care of her, but he's definitely strange. Last week he answered the door in his mother's dress. She told me he's always worn her clothes around the house and she asked me not to document this. **Should I keep this family secret?**

Nurses are asked to record detailed background information about a client's home and family when home health care is provided. There is some family information, however, that appears to have no bearing on the health and safety of the client and may pose a risk to someone's reputation and employment if it is revealed. How should this information be treated? Clearly, this situation calls for discretion. The written record should include mention of the son as the family caregiver and should document the extent and quality of the care he provides for his mother. Other observations about his behavior should not be part of the written record unless it is relevant to his mother's well-being.

Given their access to very personal information, home health care nurses should be sensitive to privacy concerns and pay careful attention to the issue of what to document. The burgeoning use of computerized records and the oversight increasingly exercised by health care insurers exacerbate these issues about protecting the privacy of information. In general, confidentiality and privacy should be protected to the greatest degree possible that is compatible with the safety and well-being of clients and others.

ETHICAL CRITERIA

- The client has the right to confidentiality, which includes the right to determine whether to disclose confidential information to anyone.
- The client has a right to privacy.

PRACTICAL STRATEGIES

When others ask questions:

1. Inform them you cannot discuss the client's health.
2. Disclose others' inquiries to the client.

When revealing confidential information to others could benefit the client:

1. Encourage the client to reveal this information.
2. Secure the client's permission to arrange a family conference.
3. Understand the legal exceptions to confidentiality.

When revealing confidential information could prevent harm to others:

1. Encourage the client to reveal the information to those at risk.
2. Determine whether the risk of harm is serious, imminent, and unavoidable.
3. Contact the agency supervisor and the ethics committee for advice.

When interpreters are necessary:

1. Try to obtain the client's permission when an unofficial interpreter is used.
2. Protect confidentiality by revealing no more information than is necessary.

When clients commit suicide:

1. Determine what the law requires.
2. Maintain confidentiality as far as possible.

When clients threaten suicide:

1. Discuss with the client the impact that the decision would have on the family.
2. Seek professional mental health services for the client.
3. Inform the client about the legal limits to confidentiality.

When the client's privacy is compromised by the presence of others:

1. Let the client decide what is acceptable.
2. Protect the client against privacy violations.
3. Discuss privacy rights with the family.

When the family's privacy is at stake:

1. Be sensitive to family concerns about revealing embarrassing information.
2. Document only what is necessary to ensure the client's safety and the safety of others.

Chapter 5

CLIENTS WHO DO NOT "FOLLOW ORDERS"

The client has intractable pain, congestive heart failure, hypertension and an anxiety disorder. Her husband says, "Whatever she wants, I do. If she wants to go to the ER, I take her." Last week they went to the Emergency Room Thursday, Saturday, and Monday. If she doesn't like one ER, they stop at another ER on the way home. Sometimes it's for pain, sometimes it's diarrhea, sometimes it's constipation. She has medications she doesn't want to take, so they play around with her medications and then run to the ER. It's very frustrating because they're jeopardizing her health. They're not managing her pain either. **What should I do?**

General Issues

- **What actions are justified when a client does not "follow orders"?**
- **What should nurses do when family care-givers do not follow the plan of care?**
- **When is a nurse justified in refusing to care for a client who does not "follow orders"?**

INTRODUCTION

The moral and legal process of informed consent requires competent individuals to accept or reject recommended treatments. Each individual thereby has the ultimate responsibility for his or her own health care choices. This responsibility, together with a growing emphasis on preventive medicine and the rise of health care consumerism, encourages people to educate themselves and, increasingly,

51

to question the recommendations and the authority of physicians and nurses. The tradition of unquestioning obedience to medical authority is still prevalent, however, in hospitals. Though hospitalized clients can exercise their rights to refuse medication or treatments, they usually consent and willingly follow the doctor's orders. People are normally motivated to adhere closely to a recommended plan of care when they have an illness or condition serious enough to require hospitalization. Moreover, once they have consented, hospitalized clients seldom have the opportunity to neglect treatment, even if they are not motivated to "follow orders" conscientiously.

Home health care clients have left the authoritarian hospital atmosphere for the sanctity of their own homes, where family caregivers or clients themselves are expected to take over the responsibility for a client's health care. In this setting families can easily become negligent and nonadherent when providing care is inconvenient, unpleasant, or burdensome for them. Once home, clients who do not want to follow a doctor's orders find it easy to postpone or skip a treatment, or to stop taking a medication altogether.

When home health care clients consent to treatment but don't follow through, nurses must contend with the ethical complexity of ambiguous wishes about treatment. They also face the professional and ethical challenge of caring for clients who thwart their best efforts to promote their health.

WHEN CLIENTS DO NOT "FOLLOW ORDERS"

This client lives in a rat-infested tenement, with trash, spoiled food, and even dog feces present. She is an insulin-dependent diabetic who is totally nonadherent with her diet. She refuses everything I suggest. Yesterday I sent her to the ER for treatment of her cellulitis. She walked out of the ER! She didn't want to be admitted to the hospital because she takes care of her grandson. **What should I do when a client doesn't seem to value her health enough to follow the treatment plan?**

Nurses usually care for clients who share with them the fundamental goal of promoting their health. For many people, their own health is more valuable than anything else. They want to live as long as they can, with the highest quality of life, and they are willing to do whatever it takes to accomplish that. They will cooperate with nurses and follow their treatment plans conscientiously. Others, however, sacrifice or compromise their own health and well-being for the sake of something they value more highly. A pregnant woman who refuses chemotherapy drugs in order to protect her fetus, a professional who neglects her own health to pursue a career goal, a man who drives himself too hard in order to earn a living for his family—all of these people challenge the assumption that good health will always be the highest value for clients.

Clients' relationships and their family obligations may be more important to clients than their own health. The client in this case, for example, values her responsibility for her grandson above any other concerns, which is an important factor to consider in developing a plan of care. In cases like this nurses should encourage clients to "follow orders" to the greatest extent that is compatible with the values and commitments that are important to them. This could require some creative suggestions to accommodate a client's family responsibilities and thus to facilitate a client's adherence to a plan of care. In order to get a client to follow the plan, nurses can educate, urge, and cajole. When the decisions clients make about their health are informed and voluntary, though, this is as far as nurses can go to promote adherence.

The difficulty in some cases lies in determining when a client's nonadherence actually constitutes self-neglect. For example, this client has significantly jeopardized her health by refusing emergency treatment for a serious medical problem. Her living conditions and her ongoing refusal to adhere to recommended dietary restrictions raise additional questions about the possibility of self-neglect. When nonadherence plainly constitutes self-neglect, questions about the client's competence also arise. Under these circumstances, nurses should inform the client's physician and the appropriate supervisor of their concerns.

> Sometimes I think we're forcing Western medicine on some of our clients. I have a Southeast Asian client who was referred by the TB clinic. He has tuberculosis and diabetes. It's hard to convince him that he needs medications. We're in there daily, testing his blood sugar, making sure he takes his TB medications and his insulin. **How can I meet my responsibilities to care for a client who rejects Western ideas about health?**

Clients may value their own health highly, but reject the standard Western ideas and practices designed to promote health. If clients do not accept the idea that what is recommended will actually help them regain their health, it is difficult to persuade them to "follow orders" and to allow appropriate nursing interventions.

In these circumstances, nurses should first of all act to assure that clients are fully informed about their illnesses and the consequences of nonadherence. Because this client could be relatively new to Western culture and medicine and perhaps has language difficulties as well, this may best be accomplished through the use of an appropriate interpreter or the cooperation of a health clinic already allied with the local Southeast Asian population. The recommendations of physicians and nurses and, more important, the reasons for accepting Western medicine, must be made as clear as possible to the client. If the client still wishes to make an informed, voluntary decision to reject treatment, that decision should be respected.

As long as the well-being of other people is not at risk, the client has the right to reject what Western medicine has to offer, no matter what the consequences are for his own health. However, if he has active TB, he must follow the treatment regimen to protect others from contracting the disease. Consequently, the appropriate public health authorities would have to be involved in that case.

My client had a heart attack at the age of forty-four. She's taking several heart medications. Now she has stomach problems, so she thinks she's toxic from the digitalis. She stopped taking the digitalis. She's been on the Internet, talking to some doctor in California about natural treatments for heart disease. She says she wants to take charge of her treatment, but I'm concerned that she may be neglecting the standard care for her heart condition. **What should I do when a client "plays doctor"?**

Clients sometimes become their own "doctors," diagnosing their illnesses and prescribing treatments for themselves. They substitute their own ideas, which can be unscientific or unusual, for the experienced judgments of nurses and doctors and implicitly reject the value of medical expertise. When clients "play doctor," nurses have the obligation to inform them of the risks of ignoring standard treatments. If clients risk their health with alternative treatments that may be dangerous or may interfere with the standard medical treatments, nurses are justified in taking a more aggressive stance in expressing their misgivings about the clients' choices. However, in the end clients have responsibility for their own health care choices, and they can reject nursing and medical judgment if they wish.

Clients can also reject the advice of any physician and seek a second opinion from another. The problem here is that the second opinion is from a doctor whose qualifications are unknown, and whose only contact with the client is through the Internet. An added concern is that the client is translating this information into treatment recommendations for her own care.

The easy availability of Internet resources encourages clients to educate themselves about diseases, treatments, and medicines, which is basically good. Generally, though, such information should be subjected to a critical appraisal and should not be the basis for rejecting standard care, without careful consideration. For that reason, the client should be encouraged to initiate a discussion with her physician about the information and treatments she has discovered on the Internet. In addition to informing the physician that the client has stopped taking one of her medications, the nurse should also express her concerns to the client and encourage her to restart the prescribed medication.

> A client in his eighties lives alone. He is a very frail man, weighing only about 90 pounds. I see him to check his blood pressure. His doctor put him on a new medication, but he's not taking any of his medications. He told me he just made his funeral arrangements. I'm wondering whether he has become non-compliant because he wants to die. **What should I do if he continues to refuse his medication?**

It is important to explore the reasons for nonadherence whenever a client will not follow the standard treatment for a condition. A client may have developed unexpected symptoms or may find a treatment regimen too taxing to follow. Nursing assessments can usually clarify whether there is a basis such as this for the client's rejection of a medication. In some cases, screening for depression may be indicated by the client's affect and behavior.

On the other hand, a competent client could exercise the right to refuse treatment in a nonconfrontational way, by simply refusing to follow the doctor's orders. Competent clients do have the right to refuse any treatment, even if that will result in death. When clients refuse to "follow orders," nurses should act to ensure that they are not depressed, that they intend to stop treatment, and that they fully understand the consequences of their nonadherence. In this case, that is especially important, because some treatments enhance a dying client's comfort. Nurses must notify the physician of any significant changes in a client's condition and disclose a client's nonadherence.

> I have a patient with a skin disorder who was put on an anti-anxiety pill for treatment. When her husband died, she stopped taking her medication. She developed the skin problem again but she won't take the anti-anxiety pill. **What should I do when a client with mental health problems will not follow the recommended treatment?**

The challenge often presented when a client is nonadherent is to distinguish a competent treatment refusal from situations where the client fails to understand the reason for the treatment, finds the medication or treatment too difficult to endure, or is not competent to make a decision. In this case there appears to be no reason to question the client's competence, thus the nurse should focus on educating the client further about the reason for the medication and attempt to determine whether there is a side effect or some other reason that the client has rejected this medication. Because competent clients being treated for mental illness have the same right to refuse treatment that all competent clients have, there is little else than a nurse can do ethically.

> My patient is HIV positive and he is not taking his medications. It's a horrible medication regimen; the side effects are awful. Now he has pneumonia. He's still drinking and using drugs, too. He's not following the plan at all. This is very upsetting for me. **How far should I go to provide care for a client who apparently isn't making any effort to improve his own health?**

Nurses have the fundamental professional and moral responsibility to establish a caring relationship that will promote a client's health and well-being. When clients continue to act self-destructively, despite serious consequences for themselves, they thwart the conscientious efforts of nurses to fulfill these responsibilities. This kind of case illustrates the frustration and difficulty nurses may face when clients are nonadherent. Their efforts to care for a client can appear futile.

There are, however, some useful strategies to pursue in this particular case, before concluding that this is futile. Despite the fact that her efforts have so far been unsuccessful, the nurse should persist in encouraging the client to seek help with his drug and alcohol addictions. Concerns about his mental health should be pursued, as well.

The nurse should also address the client's nonadherent behavior. If the serious side effects of the medication are the main reason that the client has discontinued using them, then the nurse could pursue the possibility of a different combination of drugs. The result could be a more realistic medication regimen—one which the client could follow with less difficulty. This would enhance the client's chances of a more comfortable, and possibly healthier, life. Finally, if none of these efforts work, a nurse is justified in seeking to transfer care to another nurse who is willing to accept him as a client. From an ethical perspective, no one is required to persist in futile efforts to provide care.

WHEN FAMILY CAREGIVERS DO NOT FOLLOW THE PLAN OF CARE

My client is an infant. At birth the baby had multiple life-threatening conditions and extensive brain damage, but her teenage mother wanted the doctors to do everything they could to save her. Now the girl and her mother are trying to care for this baby at home, and they are overwhelmed. I'm sure the baby is not getting all the treatments and feedings she needs. Still, if I try to get them help, they could be judged guilty of neglect and lose the baby. **What's the right thing to do in a case like this?**

When families are not providing the care they are expected to give, the first step is to address the reasons for their nonadherence. In some cases, families are limited in their ability to understand the requirements of the plan of care or have difficulty learning the skills that are needed. If that is the situation, the ethically appropriate response is to offer further education and skills training or attempt to adapt a plan of adequate care to their capabilities. Where it is not possible to adapt a plan successfully, it may be necessary to remove a client from home health care. That is the issue in this case. Though this family sincerely wants to provide good care for their infant, their efforts fall short of what is required. The most important question is what will be in the best interest of this infant. Is it better for the infant to stay at home, even with compromised care, than to be removed from home health care?

An analysis of consequences may be useful in evaluating this situation. If the benefits to be gained by removing her from the home are not likely to outweigh the trauma of separation, then the infant should be left with her family. On the other hand, when the level of care the

mother and grandmother are able to provide is so poor that it is precipitating an immediate threat to the infant's life, or constitutes abuse
or neglect, the infant should be removed from the home.

> I have a dying client who was always the controller in the family. Now he can-
> not take care of himself. The power has reversed. He complains to me that he
> is experiencing a lot of pain. I suspect his wife is not giving him the pain med-
> ications as often as he needs them. His daughter told me she thinks her moth-
> er is getting her revenge. **What should I do?**

Well-meaning families may stop following a plan of care for various
reasons. Families who just want clients to be happy could resist imposing treatments that are painful or in any way unpleasant, and they may
allow clients to enjoy habits that are now forbidden by a physician.
Still others will not impose treatment if a client objects, because they
want the client to make his own decisions and they want him to have
the dignity of controlling his own treatment. In other situations, the
family may attempt to follow the routine, but physically or psychologically be unable to make the client comply. For example, children or
spouses who are used to accepting the authority of a client may find it
difficult to insist on the prescribed treatment when a client is uncooperative. Finally, families may forget or neglect certain aspects of care
because they are overwhelmed by the role of caregiver. The proper
response in all of these cases is to renew efforts to teach the family
about the need for the recommended treatment and to seek to arrange
a family discussion to address the difficulties the family has in providing care.

Families who are actually hostile to the client they are supposed to
care for may not be sufficiently motivated to follow treatment plans
conscientiously. Nurses can address this hostility through their efforts
to educate a family about the client's illness and the effect it will have
on the client's behavior. If families understand the illness, they will
perhaps be less hostile. A discussion with the client's wife to clarify the
use of pain medications could itself solve the problem in this particular case.

In addition, there may be other ways to succeed in getting the client
the care he needs. For example, there could be other ways to deliver
the pain medication, such as a morphine patch or longer acting pain
medication, that would not rely as much on the wife's cooperation. If

a client is in imminent danger of neglect or abuse, then of course a nurse should report the situation to her supervisor and the appropriate agencies.

REFUSING TO CARE FOR A CLIENT WHO DOES NOT "FOLLOW ORDERS"

I have a client who has loads of medical problems. The real problem, though, is that she is uncooperative, irritable, and suspicious. She says things have been stolen by her aides, but she has never filed a complaint. She never has a kind word for anyone. I try not to have anyone cover for me, because every nurse who has been there came back with a horror story. I seem to be the only nurse she likes. Now she needs a colonoscopy. Her doctor wants to do this on an outpatient basis but she wants to stay overnight in the hospital. Yesterday her blood pressure shot up. I think she skipped her medicine because she thought she would have to be hospitalized. **What is my responsibility in this case?**

The issue here is whether the client's behavior warrants the termination of services by the agency or would justify a nurse's request to transfer her care to someone else. If clients are nonadherent or family caregivers fail to follow a physician's orders, the physician or home health care agency does have a legal right to end the relationship with the client. In such a case, the professional caregiver is required to notify the client in writing, giving an explanation for the withdrawal. The caregiver must recommend continued treatment if necessary, provide a reasonable amount of time for an effective termination date, and offer to make the client's medical records available to the new agency and physician, with the client's consent. Failure to meet these terms could result in charges of abandonment, resulting in tort liability. Recurring instances of nonadherent behavior or further attempts to obtain unnecessary care could justify withdrawal from the case by both the agency and the nurse.

Here, however, this nurse has been successful in establishing a relationship with a client where others have failed. She may consequently believe she has an obligation to maintain this relationship, especially if she is convinced the client is unlikely to establish an adequate caring relationship with a new nurse. The issue is essentially an issue about character. Do her own standards as a nurse compel her to continue care?

My client has chronic disease; he is very hard to manage. He's in and out of the hospital. They treat him, send him home, and in a week, he's in trouble again. It's obvious he's not following the plan. When he was admitted to the hospital the last time, the agency decided they would not take him back. They were firm. He calls the agency three or four times a day, yells and curses at everyone, he's not doing what he's supposed to do, they won't have him back on service. But this time he has heart failure, which qualifies for skilled visits. The agency has agreed to take him back. We have a contract with him that specifies that he will be discharged from service if he does not follow the plan of care. **Should I ignore any incidents of nonadherence so he won't be discharged?**

Home health care agencies commonly operate under such contracts with their clients. When two parties have a contractual agreement, either party has a legal right not to renew the contract and a moral right to refuse to renew, if the other fails to satisfy the conditions of the contract. This agency can end the relationship with the client if he does not satisfy the conditions for providing services, that is, if he does not adhere to the treatment plan.

A legal contract outlining responsibilities and rights, nonetheless, does not adequately define the nurse-client relationship. It ignores the richness of the caring human relationship that often develops between nurse and client. Thus, conforming strictly to the letter of a legal contract may not satisfy a nurse's ethical responsibility to a client.

Suppose that this nurse believes that her care is substantially helping the client, in spite of his frequent nonadherence to the treatment plan. Under these circumstances, she may be willing to continue to work with him. Yet, she is also required to keep accurate medical records, which means she cannot avoid noting any nonadherence that is significant. But if she believes the client will benefit from remaining on service, she should be his advocate with the agency and argue against his dismissal, despite his difficult behavior. On the other hand, the nurse also has moral rights of her own to request withdrawal from a hostile environment.

Because competent persons have the right to refuse treatment, clients who do not behave in accordance with treatment plans cannot be coerced. In accepting home health care, clients themselves, directly or through their caregivers, take on responsibility for their continuing care. Though nurses can appropriately attempt to persuade clients to "follow orders," there is a limit to what they can and should do for an uncooperative client. At the same time, clients have no guaranteed right to nursing care if their actions make such care ineffective or inappropriate. Agencies and individual nurses may withdraw, as long as it does not leave a client totally abandoned and without needed nursing care.

The case of incompetent clients is different, for the responsibility for care lies with the caregiver. Nurses assume the responsibility of assuring that the client is receiving adequate care. When education and oversight are not effective and the situation is serious enough, then a report of medical neglect or abuse should be made to the appropriate agencies.

ETHICAL CRITERION

• A competent client has the right to refuse treatment.

PRACTICAL STRATEGIES

When good health is not the client's highest value:

1. Ascertain why the client is not following the plan of care.
2. Educate the client about the risks involved in nonadherence.
3. Be sure that the client's choice is voluntary.
4. Encourage the client to adhere to the treatment plan as fully as possible.

When a client's nonadherence endangers someone else:

1. Explain the risks involved.
2. Contact the appropriate authorities to protect innocent third parties, if necessary.

When a client agrees to treatment, but does not follow through:
1. Identify the reasons for the client's behavior.
2. Explore modifications in the plan of care that will accommodate client concerns.

3. Make sure the client understands the consequences.
4. Propose strategies for adherence.

When the client's family does not follow the plan of care:

1. Identify obstacles that interfere with providing care.
2. Adapt the plan of care to address the problems.
3. Protect the safety of the client.

When the client's behavior raises questions about continuation of services:

1. Explain the consequences of the behavior.
2. Discuss with the client the reasons for the behavior.
3. Guarantee that the client understands the conditions for continued service.
4. Assist the client with transfer of care if necessary.

Chapter 6

RESPECTING CULTURAL DIFFERENCES

Since one of the local churches started sponsoring Haitian families, we sometimes see clients who have unfamiliar ideas about diseases and medicines. Right now I have a client who is convinced someone put a curse on her because she suffered complications after she gave birth at home. She hasn't been taking her medications because she believes they won't do any good. She's using a home remedy instead. **What should I do about her home remedy?**

General Issues

- **Is it acceptable to compromise on care to accommodate cultural differences?**
- **How should nurses respond when clients reject Western practices?**
- **Are there some cultural practices that should not be tolerated?**

INTRODUCTION

Nurses accept Western scientific assumptions about the causes and treatment of illness, but their clients sometimes have widely divergent views, attributing illness to the curse of an enemy, disturbed forces in the spirit world, or a lack of balance or harmony in natural elements. Differences in medical beliefs commonly stem from differences in cultural traditions and backgrounds. When medical beliefs are not based on Western views, they may constitute a challenge to the scientific basis for providing nursing care. They may also challenge the ethical framework of individual rights that governs Western nursing practice.

63

For these reasons, clients' cultural beliefs and attitudes about health and illness are of special import.

The moral and legal doctrine of informed consent requires respect for clients as individuals with the right to make their own medical decisions. This means respecting their individual reasons and the personal values that form the basis for their decisions. When cultural differences exist, respecting clients' values requires what some nursing organizations call cultural competence, that is, knowing and understanding the cultural beliefs and practices of diverse cultural groups. This competence is acknowledged by nursing professionals as essential to good nursing care. From a moral perspective, cultural competence is also ethically required in order to demonstrate respect for clients.

In the intimate context of the home, clients' personal and cultural values have greater significance than they would in the more impersonal atmosphere of a hospital. Hospitals tend to obscure these individual and cultural differences by imposing a protocol of treatments, standard meals, and nursing care. In clients' homes, on the other hand, clients' cultural perspectives define the very setting in which nursing care is provided. Consequently, any cultural differences that exist between nurses and clients may be magnified in this context.

ACCOMMODATING CULTURAL DIFFERENCES

I have a new client who is a Navajo. He told me he was brought up in the traditions of the Navajo community. His immune system is compromised due to chemotherapy, but he's planning on having a traditional healing ceremony. I'm concerned about his risk of infection if he is exposed to that many people. **Should I try to stop this?**

Understanding the medical beliefs and values of other cultures begins with the identification of the assumptions underlying Western medical practice, which are rarely questioned. A typical Western belief is that an important goal of science is to learn about nature in order to control it for human purposes. In contrast, many non-Western cultures instead seek to understand the natural world in order to be able to work with the elements of nature and to live in harmony with the natural order of things. For those who believe that health results from maintaining the proper harmony or balance of hot and cold elements, for instance, the choice of treatment depends on whether it will contribute to restoring that balance, rather than its possible use in the defeat of natural forces.

Another typical Western belief is that the causes of disease are elements in the physical world such as germs and viruses. A central goal of medical and nursing practice is to conquer these causes of disease, prolong human life, and enhance the quality of life by promoting physical comfort and preserving physical functioning. For those who hold beliefs that attribute illness to forces in the spirit world, however, treating the physical causes of disease may not succeed without a ceremony that is designed to make peace with those in the nonphysical world.

In fact, different cultural groups often place different values on physical health. Physical functioning and comfort could be judged less important by some cultures if the mind or spirit would be jeopardized by treatment, as in the case of a medication that depresses consciousness. Further, many religious groups place great value on a spiritual life after death. Consequently, some followers might make medical decisions designed to enhance their spiritual life, even at the expense of their physical well-being.

Though non-Western medicine has a long history, it is only recently that Western researchers have begun exploring the mind–body interaction beyond the purported and poorly understood placebo effect. Non-Western medicinal preparations and treatments such as acupuncture are also now being studied extensively and tested in laboratories. Alternative and complementary medicine has thus begun to find a place in Western medical practice. These trends reflect a growing respect for methods of healing other than those of standard Western medicine.

How can this respect be reflected in the day-to-day encounters with clients and families in home health care? It is important to recognize that a client's identity and values are defined, to some extent, by participation in cultural practices. As long as these practices do not pose a certain, imminent and serious harm, these traditions should be respected. A common dilemma, however, is how to reconcile the moral requirement to respect culturally diverse values with the responsibility to provide good nursing care. The risk posed by traditional practices cannot be ignored in cases such as the one involving the Navajo client. The best solution is to attempt to make the traditional practices compatible with the clinical advice of Western practitioners,

as far as possible. Perhaps this client could be persuaded to postpone
the healing ceremony until his immune system has been strengthened.
If that is not feasible, he might be willing to wear a surgical mask to
protect him from infection, or to limit the number of people attending
the healing ceremony to limit his exposure to germs. If he is unwilling to do this, the nurse should not support his participation at this
time.

> Currently I'm caring for a client who is a Gypsy. His house is full of people
> from his clan. They're always there, sitting in the living room, surrounding him
> when I'm trying to examine him. Asking them to leave would offend them, so
> I'm not sure what he wants me to do. **How can I best acknowledge my
> client's rights to privacy and confidentiality and yet remain sensitive to
> his traditions?**

An emphasis on privacy, confidentiality, and client's rights perme-
ates Western ideals of ethical nursing practice. Clients whose personal
lives are organized around strong social communities and complex
family networks may not place the same value on those rights. Should
individual rights be ignored to accommodate clients from different
cultures?

The appropriateness of an ethical focus on the rights of isolated
individuals is already challenged by the realities of home health care.
In this setting the client is usually best understood as an individual
with relationships, as an individual within a family, for example.
Sometimes the "family" is the whole clan or religious community. In
some cultural or religious communities it takes a whole group to nur-
ture someone back to health or to help the person make an exit from
this world. The client's well-being essentially depends on the presence
of his "family."

The community-oriented values of a client can raise concerns about
respecting client's rights. How can nurses determine whether a client
willingly accepts the lack of privacy and the violations of medical confidentiality? The nurse could attempt to raise this issue with the client
to determine his wishes if she can talk privately with him. If she is
unable to do this, she should assess whether he welcomes the presence
of others. In situations where he appears uncomfortable, she can intensify her efforts to protect his privacy. But, without his decision to
exclude other people, she must respect his right to have them there,
according to the practices and expectations of his culture.

There are lots of cultural differences that present moral issues for me. With Chinese families I've learned that I have to talk to the eldest son. I can't talk to the client to ask him what he wants to do. **How can I be certain that a client consents to treatment when the client says nothing?**

Family relationships are influenced by cultural values and standards. In some cultures, for example, gender roles and expectations require husbands to make decisions for their wives. In other cultures the young adult members of a family are expected to defer to the decisions of the oldest male in the family or to accept the decisions of a non–related elder in the community. Both the moral and legal requirements for informed consent, however, assume that competent adult clients will make decisions for themselves. Nonetheless, within communal societies, individuals may accept the decisions and wishes of the family or the group as their own. How can these cultural practices be reconciled with the moral requirement that clients be allowed to make their own decisions?

Although clients have the right to decide for themselves, they also have the right to waive their rights if they want to do so. A client can cede a right to decide to someone else, for example, his eldest son, if he wishes to do that. Determining whether someone is freely ceding a right to decide can be difficult, nonetheless, for there are no formal guidelines that can be used. Consequently, when someone other than the client has assumed the responsibility to make decisions, it is important to assess whether the client appears to agree with this, and to offer the client an opportunity to assent or dissent from any decisions that are made. In the home health care context, paying attention to the client's relationships to family and others in his community, and the consequences nursing actions have for those relationships, is imperative. For example, insisting on an individual's informed consent when it conflicts with cultural expectations could have harmful consequences for relationships that are valuable to a client. Accordingly, nurses should ensure that clients have the opportunity to waive rights, such as informed consent, if they wish to do so.

I have found that Portuguese families often do not want the clients to know how sick they are. When a family member translates, they're usually not interpreting what you're telling them. This is really a problem when a client is terminally ill. **What should I do when a client's cultural values conflict with the duty to provide full disclosure of medical information?**

The moral and legal doctrine of informed consent entails a notion of autonomy that privileges the individual over the community, as a reflection of Western cultural values. It also requires health professionals to provide adequate and truthful information to individuals, so that they can freely consent to treatment. Cultural values may conflict with this requirement to address illness directly and openly with a client.

In addition, the standards utilized in determining whether the legal requirement of informed consent has been met have an undeniably Western bias. The law has traditionally ignored the fact that some individuals either do not want certain information or defer decision making to another family member, the community, or the authority of the physician. Recently, there has been a shift toward legally recognizing the values held by individual clients and the way these values are likely to influence medical decision making. Courts have held that although objective, the standard used must consider the needs of a reasonable person with all the characteristics of the plaintiff, including idiosyncrasies and religious beliefs.

Accordingly, clients from a cultural background in which the direct discussion of disease and death is an anathema should not be forced to confront these realities, if they do not wish to do so. In cases where information must be translated by families, it is appropriate to allow clients and families to follow their own cultural practices in such matters. Nurses could suggest that families provide more information, so that a client's wishes for end of life treatment could be ascertained. But they should not reject the culturally accepted practices, unless they have good reason to believe that these practices endanger the client's well-being or the client objects.

> I have a new client, an elderly man. When I saw him, he was in bed, wearing only one slipper. I tried to remove it and he took offense. He got very upset, but wouldn't tell me why. I later found out that he's an Orthodox Jew. He is not supposed to be touched by a female who is outside of the immediate family. **Should I have known that? Is it my obligation to know details about my client's religious beliefs?**

An essential part of cultural competence is understanding the taboos that are important to people of other cultures and religions. These can manifest themselves in subtle ways. For example, clients who ask

"What's in this medicine?" could be wondering if it is made of pork products, as are some medications, or oyster shells, as in some calcium supplements, both of which might be forbidden foods.

Anyone who assigns nurses to cases has a responsibility to know some of the basic requirements and restrictions of the major religious and ethnic groups within the agency's area. A female nurse should not have been assigned to care for this client if his religious affiliation were known. If the agency had no male nurse it could assign, this should have been discussed before the agency agreed to provide home health care for this client. It might be necessary to refer a client to another agency to ensure that the client receives care that does not violate any religious prohibitions.

Nurses themselves also have a responsibility to know common religious taboos that are relevant to their nursing practice. When a client reacts unexpectedly to a gesture or comment, nurses should explore the possibility that a cultural or religious taboo has been violated and respond accordingly. A nurse should not have been assigned to this client without being informed of his religious background. The agency is at fault for putting the nurse in this position, possibly because the agency supervisor did not know the client's religious affiliation or did not understand the religious taboos that would affect nursing care.

Ethical issues arise in home health care because we are all raised differently, with different cultures and different ideas about marriage and raising kids. I do obstetrical work and have a specialization in lactation. Sometimes we are unaware of the customs. I found out that some Hmong families don't want us calling the baby "beautiful" because evil spirits might hear and steal the baby. **How can I avoid violating a client's taboos?**

The taboo on calling a baby "beautiful" would be unexpected to anyone unfamiliar with Hmong traditions. This underscores the importance of developing cultural competence. When religious or cultural taboos are a factor, the nurses assigned to a client's care should be briefed. In situations where there is doubt about the client's preferences, nurses can avoid violating unknown taboos if they explain what they are about to do and ask permission.

A word of caution is in order when considering cultural differences. It can be easy to fall into unwarranted generalizations, to assume that a person who is a member of a certain ethnic, religious or national group will share all of the traditions of that group. Yet it is important to recognize that there are individual differences. Factors such as clients' ages and the length of time in this country, whether they live within a cultural community or are acculturated, and the level of education they have attained can influence the values and practices they maintain. As a matter of fact, studies show that socioeconomic status is more important in predicting individual's values than racial or ethnic differences: middle-class families tend to think and behave more like other middle-class families than like others of their own cultural group.

WHEN CLIENTS REJECT WESTERN PRACTICES

I have a case that involves a client who has AIDS. His family refuses to let him take any of his medications. They have him surrounded by magnets. They believe "that will do it." He agrees with them; he believes that the magnets will work. **Should I go along with this?**

When clients and their families follow cultural practices, the important question is whether the practice is seen as harmful in itself by Western practitioners or whether a practice is incompatible with a physician's recommended care. Some practices, such as ingesting unknown "remedies" in place of medicines known to be effective in treating an illness, are harmful for clients. Other traditional practices could be harmless if they do not prevent the use of the treatment ordered by a physician. In some cases where there is very effective treatment, as with early treatment of breast cancer, time is lost when alternative treatments are tried. As a result, even if the client ultimately accepts therapy, the outcome is likely to be much less favorable. Nevertheless, competent clients have the right to reject Western medicine. A nurse's ethical responsibility is to exert all reasonable efforts to educate and persuade clients to abandon cultural practices that are harmful or interfere with effective treatment.

Because magnets are generally not considered harmful, the issue in this case is whether the medications which are being rejected are necessary life-saving treatments. If the client is at an end stage of his disease where medication would be only marginally helpful, the obligation to attempt to persuade him to accept Western medicine is much less stringent. Even when clients reject therapeutic treatments, nurses should continue to provide nursing care that is of benefit to the client, namely, care that promotes comfort and palliation of symptoms.

> Cambodians and the Hmong do coining; they place a hot coin over the place that hurts, and put a glass over it. I have a case where a child needs to be hospitalized, but her family practices coining and rejects the doctor's advice. **Does this count as child abuse, or are these cultural beliefs protected by the law?**

Nurses are legally required in all states to report suspected cases of child abuse and neglect. There are, however, legal protections afforded to parents whose cultural practices can be construed as religious in nature. Nearly all states have statutes exempting religiously motivated parents from being found guilty of child abuse and neglect for failing to secure traditional medical treatment for their children. Nevertheless, this case should be reported, because the child's condition warrants hospitalization. It is the role of state agencies or courts, not nurses or physicians, to decide how to apply the legal exceptions.

> Sometimes I'm not sure what to do. I have an elderly Puerto Rican client who is refusing to take her blood pressure medications. She's already been hospitalized twice. She's risking her health, but she told me she won' t take the medication because it's a "cold" medicine. She wants a "hot" medicine. **What should I do when a client rejects standard medicine?**

Caring for clients who do not follow medical recommendations is not uncommon. As in other cases of nonadherence, it is important to determine the reasons for this behavior in order to devise an ethically appropriate response. This client is rejecting standard medicine because she wants a treatment that accords with her cultural traditions. The first response then should be to ask the client's physician if there is a medication that could be used that would fit the requirements of the client's hot-cold theory of disease, that is, a "hot" medicine. Finding standard treatments that are compatible with clients' cultural ideas is undoubtedly the best solution.

When the client's cultural ideas cannot be accommodated, nurses could encourage clients to talk over the situation with their families. Sometimes a member of the family can explain the proposed treatments and persuade clients to adopt a treatment or find a reasonable compromise that successfully protects the client's health.

In the end, if a client has adequate information and competently makes a choice to reject treatment—any treatment—that choice must be respected. Whenever this is the situation, nurses should ensure that clients understand the nature of an illness and the efficacy of the recommended treatment, together with the risks of rejecting treatment. When the client has been hospitalized twice, as in this case, the consequences of refusing blood pressure medication should be clear to her. Because she is risking her life by rejecting the prescribed medication, it is imperative to exert all efforts to explain and educate her, though in the final analysis she may still refuse to take it.

> Russian families are coming in with a sponsor who sets them up in a house, maybe three families in an apartment. Right now I have an elderly Russian client with Type 2 diabetes. It was diagnosed through a screening program the Department of Health runs. It is impossible to get her to eat the proper diet. She eats her main meal of the day from one great stock pot of food that's been cooking all day. Everybody in the apartment shares the same food. She just won't change her diet. **What should I do when a diabetic is reluctant to give up her traditional foods?**

This is a common situation that home health care nurses confront when clients require special diets. People are often unwilling to change the way they have been eating their whole lives. They are especially unwilling to give up any foods that are an important part of their cultural traditions.

The significance of lifestyle changes that require giving up cultural traditions should not be underestimated. Though accepting this change in her diet may seem like a small price to pay for good health, a client may view this as an insurmountable challenge. Respect for cultural differences requires special attention to the need to develop diets that are adapted to the typical cultural preferences of clients. A nurse could negotiate with the client to develop a better diet that includes modified versions of traditional foods or perhaps refer the client to a nutritionist. Though nurses can educate, counsel, persuade, and provide appropriate referrals, there is little else that they can do. Ultimately, the client has the right to make the decision to continue with her traditional diet, even against her best interest.

THE LIMITS OF TOLERATION

> The nurses are all arguing because no one wants to go in there. The family is Buddhist. They believe you shouldn't kill anything. Roaches; won't kill them. You set up a sterile field and a roach walks across it. I told the client I need a clean place to give my treatment. **Aren't there some things that I should not have to tolerate?**

Despite the mandate to respect cultural differences, there will be situations where the cultural beliefs of clients will lead them to choices and behavior nurses consider to be intolerable. What does cultural competence and respect for differences demand? How much should nurses tolerate?

Nurses and other health care providers typically come from social, economic, and often cultural backgrounds that are very different from many of their clients. As a result, individual nurses may find some clients' lifestyles distasteful or even repugnant. Nurses may be assigned to care for clients who have low standards of personal cleanliness or be sent into homes that are extremely dirty or disorganized. Dirty environments, distasteful or repugnant lifestyles should be tolerated, however, as long as they pose no threat of harm to the client or the nurse.

There are other cultural differences which nurses should not tolerate. The clearest examples, of course, are cases in which cultural practices pose a risk of harm to the client or to others. If there is a risk of serious and imminent harm, then this must be reported to the appropriate agencies and supervisors. When a situation poses a risk to the safety of the nurse, that is a good reason to ask to be removed from the case and perhaps to suggest that the agency terminate its contract with a client.

Other cultural practices may conflict with a nurse's personal values. For example, a nurse who is a vegetarian and an animal rights activist may encounter a family whose culture recommends healing ceremonies involving ritualistic animal sacrifice. When nurses encounter cultural practices that are intolerable because they violate their personal values, they still have a duty to provide care at least temporarily, until someone else can be assigned to the case.

In this case, the impossibility of establishing a sterile field makes any treatment risky for the client. The client, of course, has the right to reject the need for a sterile field, as long as he understands the risks he is taking. But what about the nurse? Surely she has a professional and moral right to insist on the minimal conditions for meeting nursing standards for providing care. If these conditions cannot be met, she may have to recommend that the agency withdraw from the case.

Finally, there are some cultural practices that are not and should not be tolerated. For example, various courts in this country have ruled that performing clitorodectomies and scarification of minors is illegal even though these may be a common practice in certain cultural groups. On the whole, it is easier to make the case that certain practices should not be tolerated if the subject is a child or an incompetent person. When the practice is freely engaged in by competent adults, their right to decide for themselves is paramount, even if it involves what others see as doing harm to themselves. However, they do not have the right to insist on the participation of nurses or others in these cultural practices.

ETHICAL CRITERION

• Respect cultural differences.

PRACTICAL STRATEGIES

When competent, adult clients engage in cultural or religious healing rituals:

1. Determine whether the practice will pose a threat of serious harm to the client.
2. Discuss your concerns with the client, if you determine harm will result.
3. Attempt to negotiate a compromise that will diminish the risks for the client, while accommodating the religious or cultural practice.

When cultural practices limit individual clients' rights:

1. Determine whether the client has waived the right.
2. Consider whether insisting on protecting individual rights will do more harm than good.

When religious or cultural beliefs result in taboos:

1. Seek information about the preferences of religious and ethnic groups within the area.
2. Explain your nursing role to the client and ask if there are restrictions based on religious and cultural practices or beliefs.

When clients reject Western practices:

1. Determine whether the alternative treatment is harmful to the client.
2. Notify the physician if the alternative treatment or refusal of treatment is deemed harmful.
3. Educate the client about the nature of the illness and the goals of Western treatment.
4. Suggest to the physician other Western treatments that would fit with the client's cultural and religious beliefs.

When a family's cultural beliefs impact the health of a child:

1. Assess whether the child's health is jeopardized.
2. Discuss your concerns with the family.
3. Report suspected instances of child abuse and neglect.

When cultural practices hinder the performance of nursing duties:

1. Assess whether the client is at risk.
2. Determine whether the environment places the nursing staff at risk.
3. Report cases where the client or nurse is placed at risk.
4. Discuss moral objections with your supervisor.
5. Approach the agency's ethics committee for advice.

Chapter 7

FACING THE END OF LIFE

My client with end-stage cancer has finally decided he's through with all the chemotherapy. He told his sons he doesn't want to be resuscitated "if something happens." They're pretty upset about this. They don't understand why he doesn't want that. I don't know what's going to happen when he can't make his own decisions any more. **Should I intervene if his sons decide they will call the paramedics to resuscitate him?**

General Issues

- **What treatments do dying clients have a right to refuse?**
- **How should end of life decisions be made for incompetent clients?**
- **What is the nurse's responsibility to families when clients are dying?**
- **Do nurses have a responsibility to help clients achieve the kind of death they want?**

INTRODUCTION

Families who have accepted the responsibility of caring for a dying client may find the actual experience of the dying process to be overwhelming. Despite the best of intentions, they can undermine the plan of care or even neglect a client because they find it arduous and unpleasant to provide the care a dying person needs. Families can thus create problems that ordinarily would not arise in a hospital or nursing home setting, where professional staff are always on call to ensure that this care is provided.

Clients, as well as families, may feel more anxious about the experience of dying when they are on their own, without the reassuring presence of white-coated professionals. Some people prefer the security and comfort of a hospital setting to ease their fears and anxieties about dying. An apparent advantage of dying at home, though, is that it seems to allow clients to exercise decision-making authority to the fullest extent and to have more control at the end of life. In reality, they may actually have less control in this context. When a client has decided to forego heroic measures, for example, a hospital staff will respect that decision. But at home, families may panic when they face the prospect of death occurring and rush the dying person to the emergency room for treatment. On the other hand, if a client decides at the end to reverse a previous decision to forego heroics and instead seek aggressive treatment or resuscitation, this will be more difficult or even impossible to accomplish at home. More important, families are not always in full agreement with clients' decisions about life-sustaining treatment. Though they seem to accept a client's decision, they may try to impose their own decisions once clients can no longer express their wishes.

For all of these reasons, the appealing image of a peaceful, gentle death, surrounded by family and friends, is often quite different from the reality of dying at home. The reality is that home health care nurses are caring for clients and families who may be anxious, physically exhausted, emotionally overwhelmed by the difficulties of facing the end of life, and sometimes in fundamental disagreement about the decisions that must be made.

THE RIGHTS OF DYING CLIENTS TO REFUSE TREATMENT

I remember a man with metastatic thyroid cancer who was on an experimental chemotherapy protocol. The doctors didn't have any standard treatment to offer him. They were just trying to give him some hope by enrolling him in the protocol. He finally said "enough" and refused to go for any more treatments. **How should I support a client in his wish to refuse the only available treatment?**

Competent clients always have the right to decide whether to accept or reject any treatment for their illnesses, even when refusal means certain death. In a case like this one, where further treatment is futile, that is, will not reverse the progress of a disease or prolong life, there is no moral obligation either to accept treatment or to administer treatment. When clients face a momentous decision like this, what they need is information, help identifying options, empathetic listening, and assistance in articulating their own values. Nurses are often in a unique position to support clients and to act as advocates in these circumstances.

Most important, though the client has refused experimental chemotherapy treatments, he has not rejected nursing care, which often plays a significant role in achieving a good death. Nurses should aggressively advocate for all the supportive and palliative care they believe clients need. This is particularly important because some physicians tend to abandon a client who has rejected treatment aimed at curing his disease.

> There are end of life decisions that don't get addressed by the doctors. I have a young woman who has refused all treatment. Her doctor is livid: "You can live! This is nonsense!" He told me to try to get her to change her mind. But she is clear that she doesn't want anything else done. **Do I have an obligation to try to change her mind?**

In these circumstances, a nurse should first attempt to confirm that a decision to refuse treatment is a client's own voluntary decision, rather than a choice that is being imposed by a family or others. If it is clear that her decision is voluntary and informed, is it then ethically acceptable to try to change her mind? It is always appropriate to initiate discussion, identify relevant facts, and appeal to values clients hold in an effort to persuade them to undergo treatment. But once the client's decision has been confirmed as voluntary, this is as far as anyone should go to try to affect the decision. This satisfies a nurse's duty to follow a doctor's orders, even though the doctor may have wanted her to be more aggressive. It would not be ethically acceptable to manipulate the client or to attempt to dictate a decision, even if it would be in the best interest of the client.

Finally, although nurses normally have an obligation to carry out a physician's order, they also should challenge an order when it seems patently unethical. Protecting the client's right to refuse treatment, even life-saving treatment, can require nurses to support clients who have made decisions nurses themselves question. A nurse, for example, could think it is too early for a client to give up on treatment. On the other hand, a nurse may feel that a client has unrealistic expectations and is only prolonging suffering by deciding to endure further treatment. Nonetheless, it is still the client's decision to make, even if doctors denounce the decision as nonsense.

DECIDING FOR INCOMPETENT CLIENTS

One of my clients was a Comfort One patient who lived with her sister. She was being treated for complications from congestive heart failure. She understood that she could one day "crash." She made it clear she didn't want to be resuscitated when that happened. We talked it over, and I thought her sister understood her decision. But when she developed breathing problems last week, her sister called me in a panic. I went over right away. She was unconscious when I got there and the Comfort One bracelet was missing. Her sister had called an ambulance. **Should I have tried to stop the paramedics from resuscitating her?**

While individuals are still competent, they can exercise their right to self-determination by expressing their wishes for end of life treatment. A Living Will can state in general terms a person's wish to avoid the use of extraordinary means, such as a ventilator, to sustain life when an illness is terminal. Individuals who sign a Durable Power of Attorney for Health Care name someone else to make decisions for them in any situation in which they are unable to make their own decisions. For example, if an individual is unconscious and thus incompetent, the agent named in the document would have the authority to make decisions. This document can include specific instructions about which measures are to be accepted or omitted. Both of these documents, known as advance directives, carry legal weight and should determine a client's end of life care, even when the client has become incompetent. Without this documentation, the assumption is generally made that all life-sustaining measures should be taken.

Advance directives are particularly useful documents when clients are hospitalized. Home health care clients can usually forego unwanted end of life treatment by simply avoiding the hospital, because the use of heroic measures to sustain life typically requires hospitalization.

The situation is complicated if someone decides to contact emergency medical personnel when a client is dying at home. Until recently, if a family called for emergency assistance, the emergency medical technician (EMT) was required to resuscitate the client even against the client's or surrogate's wishes. In fact, even if a copy of a valid Living Will or Do Not Resuscitate (DNR) order were visible, the EMT had no legal authority to carry out the orders.

That has changed with recent legislation that permits emergency medical technicians to respect Allow Natural Death and DNR orders in the home health care setting. Comfort One bracelets, standard hospital bracelets with Allow Natural Death or DNR printed on them, authorize emergency medical personnel to carry out these orders. A request from a family member or friend does not override a valid DNR order signified by the fact that the client is wearing a Comfort One bracelet.

The issuance of Comfort One bracelets emerged as a result of a legal progression that began with the 1990 U.S. Supreme Court decision in *Cruzan v. Director, Missouri Department of Health*, which recognized a constitutionally protected liberty right to refuse life-sustaining treatment. During the same year, Congress enacted the Patient Self-Determination Act (PSDA), affirming patients' rights to refuse medical treatment, even if death would result from the refusal. The PSDA applies to all health care facilities receiving Medicaid or Medicare funds and mandates (1) documentation in the patient's medical records of whether or not a medical directive has been executed; (2) education for the community and staff on issues concerning advance directives; (3) maintaining written policies and procedures to accept or refuse life-sustaining treatment and carry out advance directives; and (4) providing patients with written information about these policies.

Following the PSDA legislation, all states moved to authorize physicians to issue "do not resuscitate" orders for consenting patients. DNR orders are activated only in the event that an individual is incompetent to express his or her wishes. These orders originally applied only to health care facilities, which included hospitals and nursing homes. Later laws were amended to include hospices and to offer "portability" between hospitals, nursing homes, and hospices. This makes it possible for the orders to remain in effect if a patient requires being moved from one type of facility to another. A licensed home health care agency now falls within the category of "health care facility" and this, in turn, applies to licensed practical nurses, registered nurses, and other health care personnel who provide services in the client's home. Thus, DNR orders are now recognized as being in force when a nurse is providing care in the home, as well as in hospitals and other health care facilities.

Most state statutes allow patients to revoke advance directives whether or not they are competent. Hence, an incompetent person may decide to revoke a DNR order, even if the decision is not consistent with the decision the client would have made if competent. Because of clients' rights in this regard, special provisions have been included in state legislation specifying procedures for notifying staff of each health care facility involved when a DNR order has been voluntarily revoked by the client. Previously, a client's revocation had to be communicated to a physician or nurse at a hospital, hospice, or nursing home. Now, the client can communicate these wishes, verbally or otherwise, to any health care personnel, who are then responsible for immediately informing the physician of the revocation.

This particular case illustrates the complexities of caring for dying clients who do not wish to be resuscitated. Though families cannot legally override a decision that a client made while competent, they may try to do so if they disagree with that decision or if they simply panic. An intact Comfort One bracelet would have guaranteed that this client would not be resuscitated by the EMTs, no matter what her sister wanted. However, once the bracelet has been removed or tampered with in any way, the EMTs are required to resuscitate, unless a physician provides a DNR order. The nurse's legal options here are limited to contacting the client's doctor to ask him to give the DNR order. From a moral perspective, she should continue to advocate for following the client's wishes when those wishes are known, as they were in this case.

> I never know what to do when I have a client who can't make any decisions. Should I just ask someone in the family to decide? That's the issue with one of my clients. She's a seventy-six-year-old demented client who is dying. No one knows what she would want us to do. **How do we decide for her?**

Proxy decision makers are allowed to make the decision to stop treatment at the end of life. It should be noted here that there is no moral difference between decisions to withhold treatment and decisions to withdraw treatment already initiated. These decisions should be made on the same basis as other proxy decisions.

If there is evidence of the client's own wishes, expressed while competent, then the proxy uses the standard of substituted judgment. This requires making the decision the client would have made if competent. Advance directives or a client's statements made in earlier conversations can be used to determine what the client would have wanted.

In a situation where there is uncertainty about a client's wishes for treatment, a nurse should ask the family about any conversations they might have had with the client about similar situations. Any relevant information from the family's conversations with the client should be documented. It is also important for nurses to document any discussions they may have with clients in which they identify their wishes for end of life treatment.

In the absence of specific instructions, when a client becomes unconscious or otherwise incompetent, nurses, doctors, and hospitals must turn to family members to give consent. There is no standard procedure for determining who the decision maker should be, though usually a spouse, partner, adult child, or a parent in the case of a young child, takes on that role. Problems can arise if the family disagrees about who should decide or disagrees about the decision itself. Nurses should encourage family discussion until agreement or consensus is reached, if possible. A legal determination of the appropriate decision maker may be needed if a decision involves life and death consequences.

If there is no evidence of client preferences, or if the client was never competent, then the proxy uses the best interest standard. The best interest standard is applied by choosing as a reasonable person would be expected to choose under the circumstances.

> I had a two-year-old with cancer. His parents knew he was dying, but they were willing to do everything that would prolong his life as long as he wasn't in pain. At the end, though, he was in a lot of pain. I still remember his mother saying to me: "Can't we just put an end to his suffering?" I gave the morphine dose that was prescribed, but I could lose my license if I gave an extra dose and I knew the doctor would not prescribe more. **Is there anything else I could have ethically done to end his suffering?**

It is clear that nurses and families should aggressively advocate for better pain management for dying clients. Numerous recent studies show that both adults and children are seriously undermedicated at the end of life, with children suffering even more than adults. Some of the reasons for this are false information about the ability of infants and young children to feel pain, skepticism about an older child's report of pain, and a fear that the use of pain medication may lead to addiction. None of these are sufficient reasons to allow a dying child to suffer.

Because he will not prescribe an increased dose of morphine, this physician is apparently acting on the basis of an accepted standard of practice that limits medication that could be seen as hastening death. A possible way to justify larger doses of pain medication is to appeal to the principle of double effect. According to this moral principle, an action that has both good and bad effects could be justified if the intention is to accomplish good, and the bad effect is a foreseen but unintended result. In this case, administering high doses of pain medication is intended to alleviate pain, though it is known that large doses of morphine will result in depressed respiration, which could contribute to an earlier death. The American Nurses' Association (ANA) Code of Ethics states, nonetheless, that interventions intended to relieve pain are acceptable even when this entails a risk of hastening death.

A good option in this case is to recommend hospice care. Clients can be admitted to hospice care when they have a poor prognosis, which is usually understood as six months or less of life expectancy. The National Hospice Organization standards state that hospice care and support is provided to enable terminally ill individuals to live as fully and comfortably as possible. Hospice provides care primarily aimed at relief of pain and control of symptoms. A team approach, including counseling, is also used to address other needs, such as psychosocial and spiritual needs of both families and clients. Clients who want treatment aimed at curing their disease cannot receive that treatment in hospice care.

RESPONSIBILITIES TO FAMILIES WHEN CLIENTS ARE DYING

I have a client, a lung cancer patient, who doesn't want to be treated any longer. His wife and sons want treatment, so he's going along with them;

they're in denial. They need to do this, and it's really making things worse. He is getting sick from the chemotherapy and wants to stop, but he doesn't want his family to know how much he's hurting. He could have a much better quality of life without the chemotherapy. He won't let me talk to them about it. **Should I tell his family he is trying to hide what the treatment is doing to him, in order to spare them?**

Clients' relationships with family members and others who are valuable and integral parts of their lives inevitably influence their end of life decisions. Clients may make certain choices or conceal information, for example, in order to maintain the status quo in significant relationships. They may fear that honest disclosures about their feelings and experiences will have an adverse impact on a relationship or they may wish to protect significant others from sadness and emotional pain. Clients' relationships are thus a crucial factor to consider when issues arise about end of life decisions.

In this particular situation, an ethical commitment to respecting a client's own decisions and his wish to control the impact of his illness on his family, supports withholding information. However, a nurse's overall obligation to a client's welfare supports telling them how much harm the treatments are doing. Does one of these commitments take precedence? The best approach to solving this dilemma is to attend to all of the dimensions of the client's individual situation, including his relationships, in an attempt to meet the ethical demands the situation imposes.

To meet the requirement to respect a client's decision, the nurse should discuss these ethical concerns directly with the client, encouraging him to find a way to tell his family his true feelings. She could offer to facilitate this discussion with his family by talking with them first in general terms, to prepare them for his dying. An honest discussion could result in his family's support for a decision to end chemotherapy.

Nevertheless, a nurse should not reveal the client's feelings about treatment without the client's approval. That is the only way to respect both his wish to protect his family and his right to determine who has access to medical information. This approach also allows a dying client to satisfy the psychological need to maintain some control over his situation.

Should the overall obligation to his welfare yield to these ethical concerns about self-determination and relationships? In fact, a comprehensive view of the client's welfare would take into account his need to have some control, his need to protect his family, and his desire to weight the consequences for his family above any concerns about his own well-being. In the final analysis, a complete assessment of this client's particular situation reveals that there is no real conflict in this case between the obligations to self-determination and client welfare.

> A client with cancer wants as much chemotherapy as the doctors will give her, even after her own doctor said there is nothing more he can do. She wants more, more, more. Her husband wants her to spend more time with their children, but she's too busy running to new doctors. He wants her to say "I've had enough." He's had enough. He talks to me about it. I don't think she believes she is that sick. She just won't hear it. **If a client's denial is hurting her family, what would I be justified in doing?**

A client's denial is not an uncommon response to a terminal illness, especially in the early stages. According to many psychologists, individuals then advance through other stages until reaching a peaceful state of acceptance of death. However, though this is a common response to death in Western culture, this should not become a prescription for how people ought to think and feel about dying. Because people have distinct personalities, values, religious and ethnic traditions, and diverse experiences with death and dying, they will approach dying in their own individual ways.

Nurses should respect a client's individual approach to dying because the right of self-determination presumably includes the right to determine how to cope with death, including the denial of impending death. In such circumstances, serious concerns that a client is depressed justify depression screening and referral for counseling. The client, however, also has the right to refuse these interventions.

The client's denial in this case and her relentless pursuit of treatment is harming her family. The resulting ethical conflict between respecting the client's wishes and protecting the welfare of her family raises an additional question: What responsibilities does this nurse have to her client's family?

Though a nurse's primary responsibility is to a client, nurses' responsibilities extend to families as well. Given the nurse's concern for both client and family, she should do what she can to facilitate a better relationship between them. Because the client may not be aware of the effects of her actions on her husband and children, the nurse should encourage a family discussion. She could also suggest the process of compromise decision making, which would provide the opportunity to address the interests of all of them. Another option is to attempt to minimize the negative consequences of the client's unending quest for more treatment. For example, the nurse should encourage the client to interact with her children in ways that do not interfere with her own efforts to obtain treatment. In these ways the nurse can be an advocate for the client's family but also respect the client's wish to approach her dying in her own way.

> Sometimes clients know what they want, but families don't agree. I had a 45-year-old client who was a dialysis patient. She was alert, oriented, functional, but she had just had it. She chose not to continue with dialysis. Her family had real trouble dealing with this. I was upset, too. I was really concerned about the effect on her family. **What exactly is my responsibility to a family when a client decides to give up treatment?**

Any competent client has the right to make the decision to stop dialysis treatments, even though the treatments are necessary to sustain life. But others may find it hard to imagine that any life-sustaining treatment is not worth the effort. Rejecting treatment, for some, is tantamount to suicide. Consequently, when clients "just give up," the effect on their families is often devastating.

If the members of a client's family disagree with the decision to stop treatment, family relationships may be seriously and perhaps irreparably damaged. Families may respond with accusations of "suicide," feelings of abandonment, and anger. The resulting bitterness may prevent the sort of personal experiences that are important to dying clients and their families.

One responsibility the nurse has in this circumstance is to help the client understand the effects on her family. If the client seems uncertain about what to do, a nurse could also encourage her to involve her family in collaborative decision making. This process may lead to better understanding and help to minimize the negative consequences when a family disapproves of the client's decision. Finally, though nurses should be sensitive to the relationships involved, they should support the client's right to make this decision, no matter how difficult that is to accept.

Unfortunately, the time allotted to a home health care visit may not allow the kind of in-depth counseling this family will need. Thus, it would be appropriate to request that a social worker become involved.

> I have a client, a widow, who is living with her daughter and her family. She has Alzheimer's. When I go into the home I see the uneasiness. Everyone is so stressed. I spend so much time trying to make peace. It is very hard. Now she has been diagnosed with breast cancer. Her daughter and son don't want her to have any treatment for the cancer because they are sure they know what their mother would want. Her granddaughter is horrified, though. When I got there today she was screaming at them. She wants me to help her get treatment for her grandmother. **What should I do when families disagree about treatment?**

Making the decision to forego treatment for a dying client is difficult. Some families respond to the reality of death by insisting on all treatment and refusing to "let go." Even some nurses and doctors who care for clients over long periods of time have a vested interest in "doing everything." For all of them, accepting a decision to refuse treatment may seem like accepting defeat. The disagreements about end of life treatment that result are distressing for everyone involved.

The key to resolving these disagreements, in this case, lies in having the family review the justification for a decision to refuse treatment. The first step is to identify and evaluate the reasons for the decision. The most compelling reason for a particular decision regarding an incompetent client, like this one, is direct evidence of the client's own wishes. Without a written document such as a Living Will, the family must rely on what their mother said at the time of her husband's death, or other comments she may have made in similar circumstances. When such information is available, the decision could be justified by appealing to the standard of substituted judgment.

If the client has not addressed the question while competent, the decision could still be justified by considering the consequences and appealing to the best interest or reasonable person standard. For any of the standard treatments, depending on how advanced the cancer is, the burdens are likely to be substantial. For a client who cannot understand the purposes of treatment, the burdens are increased. Thus, the goal of avoiding additional suffering could justify nontreatment as a good option. On the other hand, if the care would be palliative in some way, for example, removing a large mass pressing on vital organs, then the benefits might outweigh the burdens. In that case, a decision to refuse the treatment could not be justified. A review of the reasons, burdens, and benefits that can justify the decision to refuse treatment should help resolve the disagreement between family members.

Some reasons for making a treatment refusal decision for someone else are weak or frankly unethical. Decisions based primarily on the grandmother's age could constitute age discrimination, which is both immoral and illegal. Similarly, when the refusal is based simply on the fact of dementia, that refusal is difficult to justify. Likewise, if a treatment is very effective and not burdensome, such as taking antibiotics for an infection, a decision not to treat is controversial. Finally, if personal interests such as inheritance are motivating a family rather than the welfare of the client, the decision to refuse treatment can not be justified.

HELPING CLIENTS ACHIEVE THE KIND OF DEATH THEY WANT

One of my AIDS clients is fifty years old. He lives alone. His family thinks he has cancer. It is getting harder to keep the truth from them, now that he is developing multiple opportunistic infections. They want to know why he isn't getting chemotherapy. He wants me to help him tell them he is gay and answer their questions. **How much should I do to help a dying client take care of unfinished business?**

Nurses have a moral responsibility to dying clients that is outlined in the ANA Code of Ethics. The code states that nurses should act to prevent and relieve the symptoms and suffering associated with the dying process. What that means in a specific situation may not be clear. How much should a nurse do to relieve the anxiety of this client? There are limits to what a nurse should do; for example, clearly a nurse should not deceive the client's family or participate in any way in the client's deception. Thus, she should not tell them that he has cancer or provide a phony answer to explain why he is not receiving chemotherapy. She should make it evident to the client that she will not lie for him, though she of course will respect the confidentiality of information about his health.

But, now that the client has decided to be truthful with his family, there are several ways the nurse can help. She may be able to obtain written materials to help him explain his illness and could help him contact community support agencies or informal groups where a gay client can get advice and help. She could also offer to meet with him and his family to provide emotional support when he reveals the true nature of his illness. She can be expected to take these steps to help a client with unfinished business. Additional efforts would be above and beyond what is morally required.

> I've become really close to one of my clients who has ALS. We talk about death and what he wants to happen when he can't survive without a ventilator. He has made it clear that he will refuse all treatment before he reaches that point so that he can die peacefully at home. Now he has a feeding tube and we're hydrating him, but he just told me that he is going to start refusing the nutrition. I feel guilty about this, even though prolonging his life is prolonging his misery. I don't want to stop feeding him. **Do I have a responsibility to help him have the kind of death he wants?**

Nurses frequently are uncomfortable when nutrition is withdrawn, especially when the client has a feeding tube that is left in place. They may find it frustrating to be unable to provide the usual care. Relevant to this is the ANA Code of Ethics which identifies some moral ideals that establish a guideline for the care of dying clients: Nurses are to provide care aimed at fostering as much physical, emotional, and spiritual well-being as possible, in a way that maximizes the values that are most important to the client. Accordingly, in this case the nurse should support the client's decision to refuse nutrition because that will help him maximize the values he has identified. Still, some nurses believe that it is wrong to participate in treatment withdrawals designed to bring about death, even if this accords with the client's values. Under such circumstances, they might ask to transfer the client's care to another nurse on the grounds of their moral objection. The agency's ethics committee could also be consulted for advice.

> Clients who are really sick sometimes think about suicide; sometimes they tell me they want it all to be over and I know what they mean. I have an AIDS client, a man who doesn't have a soul in the world except his dog. From the questions he's been asking me lately I think he wants to know how to end his life without any pain. **What should I do about this?**

One of the most agonizing situations nurses can face is caring for a client who may be contemplating suicide. Suicide should be distinguished from a decision to refuse treatment that is necessary for sustained existence. When life-sustaining treatment is refused, death is often regarded as a foreseen but unintended consequence. The underlying physiological condition, as opposed to the client's own action, is considered the cause of death. In contrast, suicide is the intentional taking of one's own life, where the client causes his or her own death. It is important to note that death can be intentionally brought about through omissions as well as actions. In fact, it is estimated that the death of many elderly clients can be attributed to refusing to eat, "forgetting" to take medications, or "mistakenly" taking an overdose.

Nurses should question and challenge the thinking behind a potential suicide. A client could be seriously depressed or indulge in distorted thinking, in which case a nurse should refer the client for the appropriate care. Sometimes, however, a competent client may be seeking to minimize suffering and maintain control over the dying process. It is possible that suicide is rational in certain situations. Nurses could therefore face serious ethical dilemmas, torn between keeping client confidentiality and the legal requirement to alert others to a potential suicide.

Should a nurse answer questions about how to end life without pain? Should a nurse assist in a suicide? With the recent publicity about the pros and cons of physician-assisted suicide, it is possible that this subject may be brought up by a client. Assisted suicide involves participating in a client's suicide by providing the means for the individual to take his or her own life with the knowledge that the client has the intention to do so. Assisted suicide is not to be confused with active euthanasia. Active euthanasia, or "mercy killing" is the intentional taking of another's life out of considerations of mercy, for example, by administering a lethal injection.

In Oregon, the only state thus far to have legalized assisted suicide, the Oregon Nurses Association has issued a set of guidelines outlining the nurse's role related to the Death with Dignity Act.

Nurses who choose under Oregon's law to participate in assisted suicide may do any of the following:

- Provide care and comfort to the client and family through all stages of the dying process, as well as teach the client and family about the process and what to expect.

- Maintain confidentiality concerning the end of life decision the client and family make.
- Explore options with the client and family regarding the end of life decisions and provide resource information that would enable access to available resources.
- Discuss and explore the reasons for the client's decision in order to determine whether the decision is a result of a depressive illness that would preclude rational decision making.
- Be present during the patient's self-administration of the medication and during the patient's death to ease the family's suffering and provide counsel; and
- Be involved in policy development within the health care facility or community.

Nurses who choose to participate in assisted suicide may not do any of the following:

- Inject or administer the medication that will lead to the death of the client.
- Breach confidentiality of clients asking for information about or choosing assisted suicide.
- Make judgmental comments or act with prejudice in response to a client's questions or choice of assisted suicide.
- Subject peers or other health care professionals to unwarranted, judgmental comments or behavior in reaction to their decision to support and care for a client who chooses assisted suicide.
- Abandon or refuse to provide palliative care and safety measures to the client.

Those who choose not to be involved in assisted suicide have corresponding responsibilities to maintain confidentiality, refrain from judgmental comments and acts, provide ongoing care related to comfort and safety measures and comply with the law governing assisted suicide. In addition, they have the right to conscientiously object to being involved in the care of a patient who chooses suicide. The nurse must transfer care to another provider under the circumstances and may withdraw from the case only when alternative sources of care have been put in place. Nurses who oppose assisted suicide on moral grounds have the same right as those who support it to be involved in policy development within agencies and the community alike.

Although currently in most states it would put a nurse or doctor at enormous professional risk to participate in an assisted suicide, a client who asks presents a perfect opportunity for the nurse to explore the client's mental state, perception of the illness and prognosis, attitudes toward death and dying, and related topics that reveal the value commitments of the client. It may signal the need for increased pain medications, closer consultation with the physician, referral to a social worker, psychiatric counselor, or religious advisor, or honest conversations between the client and family. When confronted with this situation, nurses can ask the kind of questions that will allow clients to explore their own feelings and values. Nurses have a responsibility to listen to the concerns that families often dismiss or deny when clients are dying.

When it is possible to initiate the process, collaborative decision making may help prevent misunderstandings and conflicts in families and help clients live out the end of their lives in the way that is best for each of them. Nurses who take a role in facilitating such end of life discussions fulfill the ideal of a caring and ethically responsible professional.

ETHICAL CRITERIA

- Competent adults always have the right to refuse treatment.
- There is no obligation to provide futile treatment.
- There is no moral difference between withholding and withdrawing treatment.
- Decisions to refuse treatment may be made for incompetent clients.

PRACTICAL STRATEGIES

When a dying client refuses treatment:

1. Determine that the client's decision is free from coercion.
2. Advocate for the client's right to make the decision.
3. Educate the family about the client's right to refuse treatment.

When a dying client has an advance directive:

1. Obtain the document for the client's record.
2. Explain to the family what advance directives mean for the client's care.
3. Facilitate effective communication regarding the client's wishes.
4. Champion the rights of the client when families disagree.

When an incompetent client has no advance directive:

1. Determine whether there is any evidence of the client's wishes.
2. Make the decision the client would have made, if there is evidence of the client's wishes.
3. Choose as a reasonable person would, if there is no evidence of the client's wishes.

When end of life decisions must be made for a dying child:

1. Advocate for the best interest of the client.
2. Support the family.
3. Inform the family about available resources.

If a dying client is making treatment decisions to protect the family:

1. Assess whether this is a competent, informed decision.
2. Encourage discussion with the family.
3. Respect the client's decision.

If a dying client's denial will harm her significant others:

1. Encourage the client to accept information about the course of her illness.
2. Discuss with the client the effect of the illness on the family.
3. Suggest ways for the family to interact while the client seeks treatment.
4. Provide the family with information regarding support services.

When families disagree with a client's decision to reject life-sustaining treatment:

1. Encourage the client to discuss the decision with the family.
2. Educate the client's family about the client's right to refuse treatment.
3. Explain the distinction between treatment refusal and suicide.
4. Identify support services for the client and family.

When family members disagree about end of life decisions for an incompetent client:

1. Determine who is the client's surrogate decision maker.
2. Arrange a family conference, if possible, to encourage collaborative and compromise decision making.
3. Assist the family in coping with the implications of their decision.

When clients ask for help in taking care of unfinished business:

1. Determine whether the request falls within the scope of the nurse's professional responsibilities.
2. Consider whether complying with the request is consistent with the ideal character traits sought.
3. It is the nurse's choice to go beyond what is required.

When dying clients seek the nurse's help in achieving a good death by refusing nutrition:

1. Respect the client's right to make the decision.
2. Recognize that the client's right to refuse includes the right to forego nutrition.
3. Show concern and compassion even when there is disagreement with the client's decision.
4. Seek a transfer if the client's decision conflicts with your personal values.

When a dying client is contemplating suicide:

1. Understand what the law prohibits.
2. Assist the client in securing appropriate psychiatric care.

3. Identify the reasons for the decision and try to provide remedies.
4. Maintain client confidentiality within the bounds of the law.
5. Encourage dialogue with the family.
6. Nurses may not participate in or facilitate a client's suicide.

Chapter 8

NURSES' RESPONSIBILITIES, NURSES' RIGHTS

*I'm working on a case now where the client's son is a doctor. He overrides the medication orders from her doctor, tells me to skip doses, and then when I don't do what he wants, he complains to the agency that I'm incompetent. His mother doesn't say anything. It's an impossible situation. **Would I be justified in refusing to care for this client?***

General Issues

- **What are the limits of nurses' responsibilities to clients?**
- **What boundaries do nurses have a right to establish with families?**
- **When is a nurse justified in withdrawing from a case?**
- **What moral and legal rights do home health care nurses have?**

INTRODUCTION

Nurses have substantive responsibilities when they care for clients in the clients' own homes. Indeed, individual nurses may have even greater responsibilities than nurses who practice in an acute care hospital, for there are important differences in these two settings. The hospital setting generally provides an environment that is structured and strictly controlled by health care professionals. Hospitals can ensure high standards of cleanliness, maintain consistent schedules for care, and supervise the administration of medications. Nurses provide skilled care for clients according to a pre-established routine that is generally implemented without interference from families.

In the home setting, however, the whole environment is generally under the control of the family. Families usually administer medication, determine schedules, and provide most of the care, which must fit in with the other demands of family life. Because the family has this role, the quality of care a client receives is a more common and more urgent concern than it would be in a hospital environment. Nurses have the important moral and legal duty to alert others to these concerns, as well as the obligation to assess the safety of clients who live alone and to determine when physicians should be contacted.

Home health care nurses face all of these responsibilities essentially on their own. They are, of course, part of a team, as nurses are in hospitals, but other health care professionals are not as immediately available for advice or help with critical decisions when a crisis arises in the home. Moreover, nurses are the only ones in a position to provide a total professional assessment of the situation. In the context of these responsibilities, moral and legal issues about the duties home health care nurses have, and the rights they can claim, are compelling.

THE LIMITS OF NURSES' RESPONSIBILITIES TO CLIENTS

The client was admitted for intravenous therapy. She gets chemotherapy every three weeks; we're hydrating her after her chemo. She lost her significant other to cancer three months ago after a very difficult dying process. Soon after her partner died she was diagnosed with cancer. Now she lives alone, and she is so scared. I've tried to get her to see a counselor, which she refuses to do. She says they haven't helped her in the past. She hates her doctor and hates the nurse at the hospital. I see her every two weeks, but she's really clinging to me; she calls me every day. I'm not comfortable at all. I want some boundaries. **What limits do I have a right to establish with this client?**

Caring is deemed to be the very essence of nursing. According to the American Nurses' Association, as an example, a defining feature of contemporary nursing practice is a caring relationship that facilitates health and healing. This care orientation, according to one prominent nursing scholar, distinguishes nursing practice from other health care professions that are oriented to disease and cure.

The ideal of a caring relationship between nurse and client provides an ambiguous guideline for actual nursing practice, however. In this case, for example, caring for the client could be interpreted as giving unlimited personal attention to her significant needs, or it could be thought to require a nurse to promote the client's independence from her. In an attempt to clarify the concept, nursing scholars have identified various attitudes, responses, and behaviors that exemplify caring. Most important, caring is said to define an ethical standard for nursing actions. One nursing scholar maintains that caring provides the moral stance from which one intervenes as a nurse. Other theorists identify what is known as "an ethics of care," which recognizes caring as the essential guideline for making moral decisions. The ethics of care emphasizes what some have called women's moral voice of care, a voice of nurturing and concern for other people, their relationships, and their suffering.

The consensus is that caring is necessary for the ethical practice of nursing. But, whether caring is explained as a concern about relieving suffering, an attitude toward clients, a moral stance, or a standard for making moral choices, the concept of caring is too ambiguous to provide a sufficient guideline for making moral decisions. Nurses must also be guided by consideration of rights and consequences, attention to the particular features of a situation, the ideal of preserving valued relationships, and the goal of developing desirable character traits—what this book has called going beyond traditional ethical theory to consider context, relationships, and character.

Acknowledging all these considerations is crucial when nurses face issues about setting limits with clients, as in this case. First of all, a caring response to the client is certainly warranted; she engenders compassion and empathy for her suffering, her fears, and her difficult personal circumstances. Caring for her, however, does not require an unlimited response to her needs and demands. A nurse must set limits with an individual client who demands excessive time and attention. Otherwise, she may be forced to neglect other clients or other professional responsibilities. For example, she may find it difficult to keep her schedule of appointments, and she may be unable to give sufficient attention to the health needs of other clients. Given these consequences, the ideal of limitless caring is morally problematic. Limits can be ethically established to allow adequate attention to each client and also recognize a nurse's right to restrict intrusive demands on her own time.

Though the nurse in this case is justified in establishing these limits, she should strive to maintain a caring relationship in which she can provide support for this client. Other professionals, such as a social worker, could become involved to help address this client's needs.

Lamentably, the kind of personal attention, psychological support, and empathetic relationships that nurses view as essential to caring for clients are more difficult to achieve under managed care plans. These plans have attempted to narrow the purpose for home visits to focus on skilled nursing needs alone. Reimbursement rules utilized by managed care have become an obstacle to establishing the caring relationship that nurses have traditionally believed defines their professional practice.

> I had a private pay client, a male with a broken hip. We really hit it off. He was immobile in the beginning, but by the end of the second week, he didn't really need me. I was getting paid to hang out. He made up a schedule and expected me to fill all of it. He called and asked the agency to cancel all of my other clients and send me there. The agency did that. I told them he doesn't need me. He just wants a friend. **What right do I have to refuse an assignment I consider unprofessional?**

The nurse's function, according to the International Council of Nurses, is to assist individuals in those activities that contribute to health, recovery, or a peaceful death, activities that clients would perform if they themselves had the strength, will, or knowledge. The caring relationship that develops between home health care nurses and their clients is intended to serve this function.

Nurses' responsibilities can be the basis for determining the boundaries of a relationship with a client. This can be illustrated by considering the preceding case. In effect, this client wants to maintain a relationship with the nurse when there is no professional basis for a continuing relationship, that is, he no longer has health needs that require skilled nursing care. The nurse is justified in refusing to meet his demands because they exceed the professional boundaries of the nurse-client relationship. Moreover, nurses should generally have the right to refuse an assignment that misuses their nursing skills. The agency should thus respect the nurse's judgment that this client does not have a health problem that requires nursing care and refuse the client's demand that she keep the schedule of visits that he has developed. The responsibilities nurses have to clients are limited to the activities that contribute to the client's health. Given that maintaining a professional nurse-client relationship is the moral ideal, nurses also have a responsibility to observe these boundaries with a client.

I have a client who has been on the service for at least a year. The place is disgusting. I don't take my bag into the home because there's no clean place to put it. Her chairs are piled high with old newspapers. The client tells me to sit on the commode. She has hypertension, diabetes, multiple problems. I see her twice a week to prefill her insulin; she keeps it in a cooler because there's no refrigerator. Some days she doesn't take her insulin because she's not in the mood. Now she wants me to say she has an ear infection. I told her I can't do that because she doesn't have any symptoms. She got very angry. **How far do I have to go to meet my obligations to this client?**

Despite their commitment to the client's health and safety, nurses do not have an unconditional responsibility to fulfill every client demand for nursing care and treatment. For both moral and legal reasons, nurses must refuse any demands that are not warranted, based on their professional judgment. If a nurse does exceed her clinical authority, she may incur legal liability for the agency.

The nurse does have an obligation to contact the client's physician, in the event that her assessment reveals any evidence of a health problem. In addition, as in any case where clients do not "follow orders," she should renew her efforts at educating the client about the risks she incurs when she doesn't take her insulin. She should inform the client's physician, as well as the appropriate nursing supervisor. Also, she could refer the client for counseling and other services. Her responsibilities to the client's health and safety are met when she has taken these steps.

Finally, the ANA Code of Ethics states that nurses should provide care for clients without restrictions based on considerations of the nature of their health problem, their social or economic circumstances, or their personal qualities. Nurses should be nonjudgmental, and they should provide care without prejudice. The reality of home health care is that clients may challenge a nurse's commitment to this standard in many ways. Clients may have multiple complicated illnesses; they may be clients who "don't follow orders"; they could be hostile, uncooperative, and disrespectful; and they could even live in very dirty apartments or dangerous neighborhoods. Living up to this professional and moral ideal in this very challenging situation is a test of character.

ESTABLISHING BOUNDARIES WITH FAMILIES

Sometimes the real problem is someone in the family. I have a client who is physically incapacitated. His wife is not giving him the best care and she won't let me do my job. She asks me to do things that are harmful, then she yells at me when I don't comply. **How much do I have to put up with from a client's family?**

As an advocate for the health and safety of the client, a nurse must first assess the possible risk to the client's health in these circumstances. At the same time, it is important to consider the client's family relationships and the consequences any nursing interventions could have for those relationships. The client, for example, may prefer to maintain the status quo rather than do anything that would anger or upset his wife. That is a judgment that the client has the right to make, and it ordinarily should be respected.

In this case, the wife's instructions to the nurse and her attempts to interfere with the care the nurse provides, raise the additional question of the nurse's rights. When a family member's behavior is abusive or restricts the nurse's ability to care for a client, a nurse should have the right to establish boundaries with the family, and if necessary, withdraw from the case. In such circumstances, agencies can require clients and families to enter into contracts that specify the rights and responsibilities of both parties. Agencies have the right to terminate the contract if clients or family members fail to meet their responsibilities, as long as they give fair notice and provide the opportunity to find alternative care. This agency could establish a contract with the client that states that the agency will withdraw from the case if the family continues the abusive treatment of the nurse and interferes with the nurse's care of the client. In situations where the family member's behavior constitutes a serious risk to the well-being of the client, the appropriate authorities must be contacted.

Children can be difficult to care for. One of my clients has serious behavioral problems. He pinches me; I'm black and blue when I leave there, but his mother won't do anything about it. She's so focused on his illness that she allows him to do whatever he wants. Several nurses have refused to be involved in his care because of this. If I ask out, too, I'm afraid the agency will want to terminate the contract with this client. **What should I do?**

In such circumstances, nurses ordinarily attempt to establish limits with the child and mother. But if that is unsuccessful, as it apparently has been here, a nurse should not be expected to continue to tolerate this mistreatment. It is the responsibility of the agency to make this clear to the family by establishing a contract that specifies the responsibilities the family has and clearly states that the agency will withdraw if this mistreatment continues.

This nurse has a crisis of conscience, because she believes that the client will be harmed if the contract is terminated. She faces a moral conflict between her responsibility as a client advocate and her own right as a professional nurse to withdraw from a situation where she is mistreated. Nonetheless, tolerating mistreatment in order to care for a client goes above and beyond a nurse's professional and moral duties. She would be justified in asking the agency to assign another nurse so that she can withdraw from the case even though the result may be that the agency terminates the contract with this family.

WITHDRAWING FROM A CASE

I have a case where the client is recovering from a serious head injury. She is incontinent of both urine and stool, but she refuses a Foley catheter. She has two pairs of pants; she alternates clothing without washing it. A mental health evaluation found her to be of sound mind so she has the legal right to make decisions. She dictates what I can and can't do, but no one is willing to intervene. I can't get cooperation from her, and I don't think anyone else could either. **Exactly what legal rights do I have to withdraw from a case? Would I be risking my license if I back out of this case?**

A nursing license can be denied, revoked, or suspended if a nurse is guilty of unprofessional conduct. Unprofessional conduct includes, but is not limited to, abandonment of a patient, wilfully making and filing false reports in the practice of nursing, failing to file reports as required by law, failing to provide details of a client's nursing needs to succeeding nurses qualified to care for the client, willful disregard of the standards of nursing practice, and failure to maintain the standards established by the nursing profession. Under certain circumstances, a nurse who refuses to accept a client or to continue caring for a client could be charged with insubordination and abandonment, which is unprofessional conduct, and lose her license.

The Nurse Practice Acts outline the legal boundaries of nursing practice in each state. If charges of abandonment or negligence were to arise, these acts would be used, in part, to determine the standard of care. Each state also has a State Board of Nursing, and their regulations, along with state and federal law, contribute to establishing standards of care, as well. Home health care standards would also be used where relevant to determine if unprofessional conduct has occurred, because determining professional conduct is influenced by the setting for providing care.

Nurses must meet the objective standard of care in order to comply with the laws regarding negligence and avoid malpractice. The standard of care mandates acting as a "reasonable prudent nurse" would act in similar circumstances. Negligent behavior is that which falls below the standard of care. Malpractice is a type of negligence referring to professional responsibilities. A nurse can be found guilty of malpractice if the courts demonstrate (1) There was a duty the nurse had toward a particular patient, (2) The nurse breached this duty, (3) The patient was injured, and (4) The breach of duty caused the patient's injuries.

The client in this case is competent and thus has the right to accept or refuse treatment. However, her decisions, such as her refusal of a catheter, could make it difficult for the nurse to meet the standard of care. It is very important that nurses document incidents like this, to establish their efforts to satisfy the objective standard of care, and avoid charges of unprofessional conduct, negligence, or malpractice. As discussed in earlier cases, agencies can establish contracts that set out the requirements for continuing care. The nurse can withdraw from the case without the risk of losing her license provided that she follows the procedures outlined in the agency's policies.

I'm seeing a client for wound care three times a week. He's recovering from injuries suffered in an accident at work. Every time I see him he uses vulgar language and makes sexual advances. I have made it clear to him that this is inappropriate and unwelcome behavior, but he just laughs. If I get the case transferred to another nurse, she will face the same harassment, so I've been trying to ignore it. **What are my rights in these circumstances?**

Based on federal law, nurses have a legal right to work in an environment that is free of discrimination and harassment. The agency has an explicit responsibility to support the legal rights of individuals they employ. Thus, they should inform the client that his behavior is illegal and make clear their intention to uphold the law.

From the perspective of this nurse, the more pressing concern is whether she should withdraw from the case, given the likelihood that any female assigned will face the same vulgar remarks and offensive behavior. She has apparently chosen to subject herself to this mistreatment in order to protect other nurses. Because this kind of self-sacrifice is unnecessary, she would be justified in requesting to withdraw from the case. She should report this offensive behavior to the appropriate supervisor to ensure that the agency takes the necessary steps to avoid placing another nurse in a situation where she is harassed. The ideal solution would be to assign a male nurse to this case, though he, too, may be subjected to the client's vulgarity.

> I work in some of the worst parts of the city. I'm scared sometimes to go to certain places. The way they live, the neighborhood, the dogs. . . . One place the rats just came out to meet us. We have an escort system that goes out with the nurse if it's a dangerous area, but not all the dangers are in bad neighborhoods. I'm afraid of a client's son. He orders us around and asks us to do strange things. **Would I be justified in withdrawing from this case because I think I'm unsafe?**

The Joint Commission on Accreditation of Healthcare Organizations requires home health care agencies to both plan for a secure environment and engage in ongoing training to deal with threats to safety that might arise in the home setting. These include domestic violence, substance abuse, dangerous neighborhoods, and weapons in the home. Many agencies arrange for a member of the police or a security guard to accompany nurses on home visits to dangerous neighborhoods. Based on concerns about staff safety, home health care agencies have a right to refuse to enter into a contract with a potential client or to withdraw from care if a client's behavior breaches a contract that has been established.

Health care professionals must risk some dangers in their practice, such as caring for clients with contagious diseases. Yet there are other dangers, like providing care for a threatening client, that nurses should not be expected to face. Nurses are thus justified in asking to withdraw from cases where they believe they are unsafe. If they ask to withdraw, they must fully inform the agency about the behavior or situation that concerns them, so that other nurses assigned to the case have the information they need to decide whether to accept the assignment. Work under such circumstances should only be on a volunteer basis.

MORAL AND LEGAL RIGHTS OF HOME
HEALTH CARE NURSES

It's really tough when the doctor writes an order to stop the tube feedings for a dying patient. I think it's wrong for people to stop treatment, especially feedings, or to do anything that might hasten death. I don't want to be involved at all. **Do I have a right to refuse to care for clients who are not being fed?**

Individuals have the right to make decisions and plan their lives on the basis of their own ideas and values, without coercion from others. This individual right to self-determination is jeopardized for any nurse who is required to participate in treatment she thinks is morally wrong. According to the ANA Code of Ethics, nurses are justified in refusing to participate in care to which they are personally opposed because of the nature of the health problem or the procedures to be used, when arrangements can be made for the client's care by other nurses. Still, depending on the jurisdiction and circumstances, nurses may not be protected from termination of employment if they in fact refuse to provide care on the grounds of conscience.

Some agencies themselves may limit services according to moral ideals, which are often based on religious values. A nurse who feels strongly about the kinds of services she is willing to provide could seek employment with an agency that shares her values or at least seek an agreement to avoid assignment to certain kinds of cases.

My client has lung cancer. The doctors have not closely monitored his care; there are problems with pain control. I told them about his nutrition; they don't address this. Today I called his physician, to try to get him to see him. He was irate, rude, yelling at me: "If you're such an alarmist, send him to the ER!" He dismissed my assessment out of hand. **What can I do when the doctor disregards my nursing judgment?**

Nursing assessments and professional judgments deserve the respect of other health care professionals, but the reality is that some physicians will treat nurses as this physician has done. When a physician dismisses her nursing judgment, a nurse should assess whether the situation is sufficiently serious to require immediate action on behalf of her client. As a client advocate, nurses have the moral and professional responsibility to respond when the actions of a coworker or others endanger the client's welfare. She should raise these issues with the appropriate supervisor at her agency and discuss alternatives for getting the client the care she believes he needs.

On the other hand, nurses and doctors sometimes have genuine disagreements about the care a client needs. Physicians have the legal authority to determine medical diagnoses and to order treatment that nurses have a legal duty to carry out, unless they believe there is an error or the possibility of foreseeable harm to the client. If a nurse carries out an order that has an error or that harms a client, she may be legally responsible for the harm that results. Nurses consequently have the legal responsibility to assess a doctor's orders and to seek clarification of any orders that seem questionable. Decisions to refuse to carry out physicians' orders should be fully documented.

Because nurses also have a legal responsibility to perform nursing assessments and communicate those assessments to the physician, it is also important to document the events when a physician rejects a nurse's assessment of a client's condition. If a physician or hospital were sued for malpractice, the question of whether the nurse kept the physician informed could be a central issue.

> My client has had three strokes in the last year. The doctor told her: "You won't get any better. There's no real potential for any improvement. You should be in a nursing home." He was so cold and brutal when he talked to her. All her therapists disagreed with her doctor. But the agency agreed and pulled everyone out of the home. **What rights do I have when I disagree with the agency's decision to discharge a client?**

Nurses are bound by contractual obligations to their employer agencies and to their clients, as well as being legally obligated to follow physicians' orders unless an error has been made or harm may be done to the client. Apart from these circumstances, nurses appear to have no legal right to act contrary to physician or agency decisions. From a moral perspective, however, this nurse could advocate with the agency and the physician to attempt to get the client the services she believes she needs in the home setting the client desires.

Once people are out of the hospital, their doctors don't want to hear about it. There was one lady who had cancer with extensive metastases. I'm surprised she's still alive. I saw her two days after she got out of the hospital. She was not feeling well; she had low blood pressure; she was orthostatic. I called her doctor, but he wouldn't order anything. He said: "How well do you know her? She's a complainer." I argued with him: "Her numbers speak for themselves: 70/40 when she stood up. Take her back and rehydrate her." He wouldn't do it. **What's my responsibility as a client advocate in this case?**

Given her extensive disease and poor prognosis, the doctor's failure to respond to the client's low blood pressure may not harm her long-term interest. If the dehydration were addressed, though, the client would probably be more comfortable. But, despite her efforts, this nurse has been unable to convince the physician to do that. Do nurses have a responsibility to do anything more to secure treatment that could make a client more comfortable?

Because there is no overt need to protect this client from the harmful actions of others, there is no legal obligation to pursue this further. A nurse may feel she should do more, however. This is primarily an issue about character and the moral imperative to meet the ideals of good nursing practice. Instead of simply accepting this doctor's response, the nurse could actively seek a way to help her client. She could, for example, discuss this with the client and appeal to the appropriate supervisor as an advocate on behalf of her client. Because the necessity of providing this care has been disputed by the physician, there may be little more that she can do.

However, given that home health care nurses have the responsibility of providing a nursing assessment of a client's condition, she could urge the agency to develop a policy that would guarantee timely access to physicians to convey assessments and clinical information and to request further evaluation of clients. She could also ask the agency to consider adopting an appeal process that nurses could use in these circumstances to facilitate consideration of issues about client care.

Based on widely accepted moral standards, nurses have certain rights they can legitimately assert. These rights include the right to be treated with respect and dignity, the right to equitable pay and reasonable work schedules, the right to work in an environment that is free of discrimination and harassment, the right to practice in a safe environment, the right to consult other professionals as necessary in the performance of their professional duties, the prima facie right to act on the basis of conscience, and the right to transfer care to another nurse when one of these rights is violated. In practice, nurses often waive these rights out of conscientious concern for their clients.

Nurses' moral rights have not received sufficient attention in discussions of the practice of nursing. As the health care system changes and professional nurses are accorded more responsibility and greater respect, local and national nursing organizations will be more successful in educating the public and other health care professionals about nurses' rights.

ETHICAL CRITERIA

- Nurses have a responsibility to serve as a client advocate.
- Nurses have a right to set boundaries with clients and families.
- Nurses have a right to be treated with respect and dignity.
- Nurses have a right to work in an environment free from discrimination and harassment.
- Nurses have a right to practice in a safe environment.
- Nurses have a prima facie right to act on the basis of conscience.
- Nurses have a right to transfer care to another nurse in cases when rights have been abridged.

PRACTICAL STRATEGIES

When clients' demands exceed the bounds of professional responsibility:

1. Determine whether meeting these demands would interfere with other professional responsibilities.
2. Establish limits with the client, as needed.
3. Refuse requests that conflict with professional and legal standards.

When families interfere with care:

1. Discuss the problematic behavior with the family.
2. Have the agency establish a contract with the client that outlines expectations concerning conduct.

When a nurse finds a client's behavior distressing or threatening:

1. Discuss concerns with the supervisor.
2. Enlist the help of a social worker, if possible.
3. Have the agency establish a contract with the client to outline the limits of conduct.

When a nurse cannot in good conscience do what is asked:

1. Contact the supervisor.
2. Arrange for another nurse to take over the care of the client.

When a nurse disagrees with a physician's orders or treatment of a client:

1. Advocate for getting the client the needed care.
2. Discuss with the appropriate supervisor.
3. Contact the agency ethics committee, if one exists.

Chapter 9

CARING FOR CLIENTS WITH
MENTAL ILLNESS

It's the landlords who take care of so many of these clients who live alone. I have an elderly client with dementia who is hallucinating. Last week he thought the place was burning down. He was knocking on people's doors in the middle of the night and trying to drag them out of their apartments. His landlord called me to say, "Isn't this man a client of yours? You better do something. He shouldn't be living alone." **What rights does a client have in these circumstances?**

General Issues

- **What are the rights of clients with mental illnesses?**
- **What is the client advocacy role of the psychiatric nurse?**
- **What special responsibilities do nurses have when clients have mental illnesses?**
- **When is mandatory treatment justified?**

INTRODUCTION

The environment in which a client resides may have a significant impact on the success of treatment for an illness. When clients with mental illnesses are hospitalized, their psychiatrists and nurses are in a position to virtually ensure that the environment is a structured one, free of disturbing distractions and conducive to effective treatment. By contrast, in the home setting the environment cannot be controlled to the extent that might be desirable from the perspective of professional caregivers. Clients consequently may receive care that falls short of the ideal treatment for their mental illnesses.

A second important factor in many cases of mental illness is the role that families and relationships have played in the client's life. A client's illness may in fact be due to mistreatment as a child or to violence suffered within a close relationship, or a client may have a substance abuse problem that is exacerbated by tensions within a family. Within the hospital setting a client's contacts with those individuals who contribute in some way to the client's difficulties can be strictly controlled. Also, a client who is dangerous to self or to others can be carefully monitored and, if necessary, placed in a locked inpatient unit. These options are not available when clients are treated for mental illness in the home setting. Determining whether a psychiatric crisis exists that requires emergency treatment in a hospital setting is one of the daunting responsibilities for nurses.

Home health care nurses most commonly care for clients with mental illnesses when clients suffer from a persistent, severe mental illness, or they have both a medical problem and a mental illness. Most psychiatric home health care focuses on managing medications, which are frequently prescribed for use on an "as needed" basis, and evaluating the need for hospitalization of clients in the event of a crisis in their illness. These responsibilities are faced in circumstances where nurses may find it challenging to establish a successful nurse-client-family relationship as a basis for providing nursing care. Moreover, home health care nurses must cope with special concerns about their own moral and legal responsibilities when their clients are vulnerable to exploitation or mistreatment, threaten the safety and welfare of others, or demonstrate impaired judgment.

RIGHTS OF CLIENTS WITH MENTAL ILLNESS

I'm always concerned about the safety of my clients. I have a young mental health client who lives on the third floor of an old house. This is a good apartment for him. He can't tolerate public housing because he can't tolerate people around him. The problem is that there is a crack house on the first floor. When he comes home there are usually a couple of addicts hanging around, sitting on the front steps. They ask him to pay money to get into his apartment, and he does it. I'm worried that this will escalate, but he prefers to put up with this. He doesn't want me to call the police. **Should I do something about this, even though he disagrees?**

Clients with mental illnesses may be particularly vulnerable to exploitation by other people. Consequently, nurses and families are often tempted to intervene in their lives, for their own good. However, unless a client is incompetent, or a client makes decisions that are uninformed or involuntary, such paternalism cannot be justified. As is true for competent clients generally, mentally ill clients who are competent have the moral and legal right to make their own decisions about where they will live and the risks they are willing to take. In this case, the client's decision to acquiesce to requests for money is apparently voluntary and informed. There is no evidence that he has been explicitly threatened or that he has been physically coerced into making that decision. Of course the nurse should monitor the situation to assure herself that he continues to prefer this living situation over his other options and that he has not been forced to agree to these requests. She can appropriately use persuasion and education to address her concerns with her client, but paternalistic intervention would not be justified.

It is important to note that remaining in a housing situation that is not safe does not necessarily signify incompetence. Even mentally ill individuals who choose to live on the streets are not, on that basis, considered incompetent. Many clients, indeed, report that they feel safer on the streets than in shelters or institutions. Thus, remaining on the streets under these circumstances or deciding to live in unsafe housing should not be regarded as sufficient to warrant paternalistic intervention.

This case also raises questions about the responsibilities nurses have when clients report illegal behavior. If this nurse has evidence that illegal drug activity is taking place in this house, she faces an issue about character: What is her responsibility as a citizen? What are her responsibilities to public health and safety? Do these responsibilities override the obligation to respect a client's wishes? If she decides to report her suspicions to the police, she should do so without revealing information about her client's encounters with his neighbors, given his wish to remain silent about this.

I have a client who is a schizophrenic. Now he is hearing voices so his psychiatrist changed his medications. His wife told me, "He won't take this if he knows it's for the voices." **Should I volunteer the information if he doesn't ask?**

Mentally ill clients who are competent have the right to give or withhold informed consent to treatment, based on the right to self-determination. However, valid consent can only be exercised if the client is provided with adequate and truthful disclosure of the treatment options, together with the risks and benefits of each option. The fact that clients may be cognitively impaired, suffering from a mental illness, or diagnosed with a substance abuse problem, may complicate the provision of information that is relevant to an informed decision about treatment. For that reason, nurses and physicians must develop appropriate information that can be provided in a way that is responsive to the needs of the mental health client. Clients should not in any case be deceived about the medications they are receiving, no matter how great the risk is that they will refuse to take them.

In this situation, the nurse should fully inform the client about his new medication, whether or not he specifically asks what the drug is. Perhaps he will consent to take this new drug if he is educated further about the reasons for the change in medications and the goals of this treatment. Nevertheless, as long as he is competent, he has the right to refuse this medication, as well as any other treatment for his schizophrenia, unless treatment has been mandated by a court order.

Informed consent to treatment is usually explicit. In some cases, though, clients give their implicit or implied consent simply by being cooperative. This, too, constitutes valid consent. Clients also give their implied consent in situations where they make no objection to a procedure, either when the nurse asks permission or when she prepares to begin a procedure. In the latter case, especially with clients whose psychological or cognitive limitations make them vulnerable, nurses must be sure clients appreciate the fact that they can object if they wish.

I had a referral for an assessment of a client's mental health status. His private duty nurse met me at the door. She said, "Can you see him, but not tell him why you're here? I think it might upset him." **Would it be wrong to assess his mental status first, then decide what to tell him?**

Therapeutic privilege is the claim that withholding information is justified because disclosure would hinder treatment, pose a risk of psychological damage to the client, or render the client incapable of making a rational decision. This may be thought to justify the assessment of mental health status without obtaining informed consent, in order to avoid upsetting a client. The claim of therapeutic privilege, though, should always be scrutinized carefully. Only convincing evidence of a clear risk of such harm would justify the failure to disclose the purpose of an assessment and the failure to seek informed consent.

A client should not be assumed to be incapable of consenting to a mental health evaluation. Though an individual may not be competent in a particular area, such as financial matters, he or she might still be competent to make decisions about specific medical treatments. In fact, a client's competence to make a particular medical decision should be assessed independently of his or her competence to make other choices, at the time a decision is required.

In this case, it would be wrong to assess this client's mental health status without his permission. As a competent client, he should be asked to give his informed consent, which he cannot do if he lacks the relevant information about the purpose of the nurse's visit. His cooperation with an assessment cannot be construed as implicit consent, either, in those circumstances. Assessing the mental health status of clients without consent can only be justified if there is evidence that the client is so severely impaired that he or she is not competent to give informed consent for any treatment or evaluation. In that event, permission should be sought from a surrogate decision maker.

> I have a male client in his early twenties who is living with his parents. He suffers from a major mental illness. His mother understands that he needs help, but his father doesn't believe there is anything wrong with him. He doesn't believe his son should be on medications. The father tells him, "You're not going to take this." Then he told me, "He doesn't need this. He'll snap out of it if you just leave him alone." **What role should his family have in these decisions?**

Families often make decisions for clients with mental illnesses, even when clients are competent and should be allowed to make these decisions themselves. Clearly, nurses must support the client's right to decide when families attempt to interfere in this way. At the same time, this nurse can encourage the family to discuss together the options the client has and their concerns about his treatment and his illness. Clients and families could use collaborative or compromise decision-making processes when decisions about care and treatment must be made that will affect all of them. The final decision, nevertheless, remains with a competent client. This client should thus be the one to decide whether he takes medication for his illness. His father should not be allowed to veto his son's decisions.

The father's comments reveal that he may not accept the prevalent theory of mental illness that governs the treatment for his son. The prevailing medical model holds that many, if not all, mental illnesses have a biological basis or cause. According to this model, mental illness is parallel to physical illness and should be treated in similar ways. Psychotropic drugs and physiological treatments such as biofeedback are thus appropriate and effective methods for treating such illnesses. Instead of accepting the idea that mental illness has a biological basis, though, some people view mental illness as a kind of moral failing that can be controlled by effort and will power. Medications are sometimes considered unnecessary or a sign of moral weakness. This is apparently the view of the client's father who thinks his son can "snap out of it."

In response, the nurse should increase her efforts to educate the client's family about his illness and the need for psychiatric medications. If the client's father attempts to prevent his son from taking the prescribed medications, it may be necessary to report this to the appropriate authorities.

> There are a lot of family issues. I have a twenty-two-year-old client, a schizophrenic, who is living with his parents. They were giving him his medications for a while, then they stopped because of the side effects. As a result he became disruptive, pacing at night, swearing at his father, and washing his hands obsessively. They started his medications again for a few days, but now his parents have decided they don't want him on any medication. It turns out that they are philosophically opposed to medicating clients for mental illness. They asked me to help them get him committed to a psychiatric facility. **What should I do if I disagree with his family about what is the best treatment for him?**

It is important, first, to determine whether this client chose to stop taking his medications, which of course is his right. On the other hand, if his parents have unilaterally decided to withhold his medications, they are interfering with the physician's recommended treatment and endangering his health. If she cannot convince his parents to restart his prescribed medications, the nurse should immediately report this to the appropriate nursing supervisor and the client's physician.

In the past, families could rather easily have a family member committed involuntarily to a psychiatric facility. That began to change with the passage of the Community Mental Health Centers Act of 1963, which had as its goal the deinstitutionalization of psychiatric clients. This act, together with federal legislation establishing benefit programs that covered individuals with a mental disorder, and changes in laws that made involuntary hospitalization more difficult, led to the release of large numbers of hospitalized patients to live in the community. These social policies, conjoined with a growing emphasis on clients' rights, resulted in the establishment of the legal mandate to provide treatment that is the "least restrictive alternative." This requires that appropriate and effective treatment for mental illness be provided in the least restrictive setting. The restrictiveness of the treatment setting is evaluated in terms of the limits placed on physical freedom and the range of activities available to the client. Halfway houses and total institutions like psychiatric hospitals impose greater restrictions that vary depending on the use of physical restraints, the amount of supervision, whether unsupervised private bathroom visits are permitted, and whether the client is conferred adult status, which is signified by allowing a locked bedroom.

Because this client can receive effective treatment for his illness in his parents' home, he has a moral and legal right to continue with treatment in that setting or a comparable one, rather than the more restrictive setting of a psychiatric facility. If his parents are unwilling to cooperate in the prescribed treatment for his illness, the nurse should advocate for his placement in another setting that would constitute the least restrictive alternative. Clearly she should not agree to help his parents have him committed to a psychiatric facility.

> I have a client who has bipolar illness that has not been controlled with medications. Recently he developed a serious medical problem and called me. I told him to call the paramedics; I was on the way. The problem was that he did not give me permission to share any information with the medical people. Can I say, "Don't transport him without restraints. He will try to jump out"? **How can I decide how much information I would be justified in sharing under these circumstances?**

Based on the right to self-determination, clients have the right to confidentiality and thus the right to control access to information about their health. This is especially important for clients who have psychiatric diagnoses or substance abuse problems, given the stigma that has historically attended these illnesses. Such information can normally be disclosed to other health care providers only if the client has signed a release granting permission to share information as required to protect his health and safety. In these circumstances, however, the nurse appears to be justified in informing the paramedics of the serious risks to her client if he is sent to the hospital by ambulance, even without his permission.

Confidentiality can be justifiably breached on the grounds that it is necessary to protect the client from serious, imminent harm. The decision about how much information to share should be governed by the condition that disclosure be limited to the minimum that is required in order to treat him effectively and safely.

> I have a client who has been hospitalized multiple times for treatment because he is nonadherent with his medications. He is a chronic manic depressive. When he's manic he is the nastiest, most vicious person I ever met. He now has court-ordered mandatory treatment. I see him once a week to give him an injection of prolixin decanoate. He tells me, "I don't want it." **What rights does he have if he is receiving mandatory treatment?**

Nonadherence is a recurring problem with many clients who have a mental illness. Because the side effects of most psychiatric medications are difficult to tolerate, clients may stop taking medications as soon as their symptoms improve. Unfortunately, their illness may significantly worsen before they or others recognize that they need help. Nonadherence with medications is, in fact, the main cause of relapse and rehospitalization for clients with mental illnesses. Nurses thus have a particularly important obligation to teach clients about the need for psychiatric medication and to monitor their adherence to prescribed treatments.

Because this client has court-ordered mandatory treatment, he obviously does not have the right to refuse the treatment. However, he does have rights of confidentiality and privacy. Both voluntary and involuntary clients retain the legal right to confidentiality of medical records, as well as the right to privileged communication. The latter is a subcategory of confidentiality referring to the statutory protection from disclosure of incriminating information revealed in the context of certain professional relationships. In *Jaffe v. Redmond*, the U.S. Supreme Court affirmed that a therapist need not disclose the content of therapy sessions even in a court of law. This protection has been extended in some states to the nurse-client relationship.

However, there are exceptions to both privileged communication and confidentiality. The *Tarasoff v. Board of Regents* court decision found that health care professionals have a legal duty to warn of harm to specific others, as well as a duty to warn of threatened suicide. The duty to warn has become the standard of care, following the requirements established by that decision.

THE CLIENT ADVOCACY ROLE

My client is a young woman who is a schizophrenic. She is also retarded. Her mother is taking care of her. I want this woman to learn to read and to have some training so that she can work. Her mother said, "She can't work." She confided she doesn't want her daughter to leave the house, and she doesn't want her to be near any men. She also told me she is concerned about losing the SSI check if her daughter works. I think her daughter would benefit from these programs. **What should I do when the mother's decision is not in her daughter's best interest?**

When a client is not competent to make decisions, a family member normally is recognized as the surrogate decision maker, an arrangement that can be formalized through the appointment of the family member as a legal guardian for the client. Surrogates should make decisions for clients on the basis of substituted judgment when it is possible to know what the client values and what decision he or she would make if able to do so. Where that is not possible, the standard of best interest must be used.

In this case the surrogate decision maker has made a decision that is apparently against the best interest of her daughter, because a program that provides training and employment opportunities would assuredly offer several long-term benefits. On the other hand, the client's participation in programs outside the home against her mother's wishes may adversely affect her relationship with her mother. These various benefits and costs should be weighed carefully to determine the client's best interest, taking into account the client's wishes and values, to the extent they can be ascertained. If the nurse concludes that the overall best interest of the client is served by enrolling her in this program, she should discuss this further with the client's mother and attempt to convince her to agree to her daughter's participation. The mother's refusal may mean the nurse should raise her concerns about the client with the physician and her supervisor at the agency. In cases where the best interest of a client is seriously at risk and it is necessary to act to protect the client, the nurse should alert the appropriate authorities. A guardian or conservator should be sought through legal proceedings.

Finally, the client's mother has decided to limit her daughter's social interactions and clearly intends to keep her at home, away from men. These decisions may violate her daughter's rights. Relevant here is the *Foy v. Greenblott* court decision, which established that every psychiatric client has the right to individualized treatment under the least restrictive conditions feasible, posing minimized interference with a patient's individual autonomy and social interaction. As a consequence, clients with mental illness who are institutionalized have the right to privacy and personal association, which includes the right to have consensual sexual activity. Home health care clients presumably have the same rights.

> The problem I have is with physicians who don't want their clients to see a psychiatrist. They tell the client, "You don't need a psychiatrist. I'll prescribe something for your depression." They address the symptoms, but they don't try to solve the basic problem. **What is my responsibility when this happens?**

The nurse's primary commitment is to the health, well-being and safety of the patient, according to the American Nurses' Association Code of Ethics. In general, then, nurses have a responsibility to advocate for access to specialists and services that they believe serve the best interest of the client. This is particularly important for clients with mental illness, who are often subject to biased treatment, and who may be unable to advocate effectively for themselves.

Clearly in a case such as this one, where a client would benefit from diagnosis and treatment by a specialist, nurses have the responsibility to advocate for referral to a psychiatrist. Unfortunately, getting clients access to care for mental health problems may be so difficult under some managed care plans that having an internist prescribe medication is the best option available.

> I have a client who keeps showing up at the emergency department with a complaint of shortness of breath and difficulty breathing. Her doctor is ignoring these complaints because she has a diagnosis of anxiety. I'm concerned that she may have chronic obstructive pulmonary disease. **What is my responsibility as a client advocate?**

Whenever a nurse has entered into a contract of care with a client, she has a moral and legal duty to act in the interest of the client. According to the ANA Code of Ethics, the nurse must take appropriate action if the rights or best interest of the patient are jeopardized by the practice of any member of the health care team. At times, a nurse must intervene in order to protect the client. Nurses must also be capable of effectively communicating the basis and urgency of various needs of a client to other health care professionals. This is particularly important because nurses can be held legally responsible for the care provided by others under certain circumstances.

In this case the nurse should discuss the client's symptoms with her physician and communicate her concerns about COPD as clearly and as forcefully as she can. She can also talk to the client about her complaints and urge her to seek a second opinion about her illness. Finally, if a physician or other professional caregiver does not provide adequate care for a client, a nurse's responsibility is clear. She should express her concerns directly to the physician or caregiver, and, if necessary, contact the appropriate authority. She should also report to her supervisor at the agency with her concerns about inadequate care.

SPECIAL RESPONSIBILITIES

> I have an Hispanic client with post-traumatic stress syndrome. Recently he has started seeing a cultural healer who dispenses herbal treatments. My client said it's for the spirits. He doesn't think he needs any other treatments. I'm worried that he will take too much of these herbal treatments. Who knows what that will do to him? **Should I ask his physician to have treatment mandated, to protect him?**

Cultural competence is particularly important when caring for clients with mental illness, because some cultures deny the existence of mental illness or attribute mental illness to spiritual forces. Nurses should be familiar with the specific beliefs of a client's cultural group, as well as the symptoms that are commonly attributed to culturally specific syndromes. Cultural competence will also help nurses understand the attitudes of families and community caregivers when clients suffer from mental illness. Although nurses should advocate for effective, safe treatment, they should attempt to accommodate cultural beliefs concerning mental illness.

In some cultures, mental illness is thought to have religious significance. Some traditions associate mental illness with negative forces, such as Satan, or see it as punishment for sin. Others place the blame for the illness on the evil eye, a curse or a hex. In such traditions, the mentally ill are often avoided or even banished. Other traditions see the person who exhibits unusual thought patterns or behavior as chosen by God, someone who is to be honored and protected. The phenomena of speaking in voices, trancelike conversion experiences, and extreme emotion may be recognized as important expressions of religious fervor. In any of these traditions, the treatments of Western medicine are believed to be ineffective and unnecessary responses to mental illness.

Of course the client in this case has the right to make the decision to use herbal treatments instead of the prescribed treatment for his illness. The nurse should fully inform him of the risks of herbal treatments, including the possibility that his condition will worsen significantly. Nevertheless, because there is no evidence that the client is clearly dangerous to self or to others, there is no basis for asking the physician to seek court-ordered treatment. It would be an unjustifiable paternalistic intervention to seek treatment for the client's own good in this instance.

> I'm concerned about my clients' safety all the time, and I mean all the time. I cross my fingers and hold my breath that the way I left them will be O.K. until I can get back for my next visit. I am seeing a client who has been suicidal. She is on medication for anxiety, and I am there to monitor her medications and assess her mental health status. With suicidal clients there is always the fear factor. I wonder if I can trust them and if they will tell me if they have suicidal thoughts. **How do I know the client is telling me the truth if she says she is fine and doesn't think about suicide anymore? What is my responsibility in this case?**

Nurses have the professional and moral obligation to assess clients with mental illness for the need for hospitalization. In order to assess a client's mental health, though, a nurse must rely to a large extent on what a client tells her. Clients who lie or withhold information complicate the assessment of their health, particularly the assessment of the risk of suicide.

In general, clients who are at risk of committing suicide present several challenges for a psychiatric nurse. They may refuse to cooperate meaningfully in assessment and treatment, they may be nonadherent with their medications, and they may conceal their thoughts of death or suicide.

When dealing with suicidal clients, nurses have several specific responsibilities. The nurse's first responsibility in such cases is to assess the client's mental health and the threat of suicide carefully and to seek hospitalization if necessary. Second, nurses have a legal duty to warn and must take action to protect a client and others threatened with harm. Third, they must disclose a client's intention to commit suicide or to harm others to other professionals involved in the care of the client. Finally, nurses must document these concerns and any measures they have taken to reduce the danger.

Though these issues may arise with clients with terminal illnesses who are clinically depressed and perhaps suicidal, it is not as common for psychiatric nurses to be involved in the care of clients who are terminally ill. These clients are usually getting psychiatric home health care only if they are already being treated for mental illness when a terminal illness develops, in which case one nurse usually provides both medical and mental health care. They may also receive mental health services if hospice becomes involved, because hospices have mental health providers.

MANDATORY TREATMENT

My client has a horrible abuse history. Her father sexually and physically abused her. She had his baby when she was fifteen. He took the baby from her as soon as it was born, and she never saw the baby again. She has constant flashbacks, and she is full of hatred and anger; she especially hates men. She is horrendously suicidal. I don't think she will ever do it, but I'm not sure. That's what bothers me. **How certain should I be that a client is dangerous to herself to justify a recommendation for mandatory treatment?**

Although most mentally ill clients voluntarily seek medical help, some clients are subject to involuntary treatment. Involuntary treatment takes place when a client has the legal capacity to provide consent for psychiatric care but nevertheless refuses care. When such individuals are deemed a danger to self or others, their treatment is mandated and thereby becomes involuntary. This may include hospitalization, but it could mean that a client receives court-mandated treatment as an outpatient. Nurses have the responsibility to assess whether the circumstances of a particular client present such a risk, given that they have a duty to intervene in such situations.

With clients who may be suicidal, the difficulty is in judging whether suicide threats are credible and thus justify mandatory treatment. The moral difficulty arises from the conflict between a competent client's right of self-determination, which assigns decisions about treatment to the client herself, and the best interest of the client, which may require treatment against her will. Mandatory treatment is a serious move that should not be undertaken lightly, even though it is aimed at preventing harm to a client. In the nurse's professional judgment this client will not commit suicide, but she is not completely confident about her judgment. Would she be justified in recommending mandatory treatment in such circumstances of uncertainty? The agency's ethics advisory committee could be consulted for advice and help in weighing the pros and cons of alternative actions in this case. Of course, nurses should carefully document their concerns and any actions they have taken and notify the supervisor and the client's physician of these concerns.

> My client had previously been treated for an anxiety disorder that was diagnosed after she expressed suicidal thoughts. Two weeks ago she gave birth to a daughter. Her husband moved out soon after she came home from the hospital. I went to her home to do an assessment. I was interviewing her, the house was dark, she said, "I'm losing it." I'm concerned about postpartum depression under these circumstances but the client is worried that if she agrees to treatment she will lose custody of her daughter. Then she confided that she is a witch. **Should I push for mandatory treatment?**

In the home health care setting, involuntary treatment is often a result of a client's inability to recognize the seriousness of the illness, for instance in cases of anorexia nervosa or court-ordered treatment following a Driving While Intoxicated conviction. It is possible that this new mother is not fully aware of the seriousness of her depression or the risk of harm to the infant.

The nurse needs to do a close assessment of the situation. If in her judgment, there is serious risk to the infant, she has a duty to notify the child protective agency and recommend immediate removal of the infant. That will result in at least a temporary loss of custody, but the nurse really has no choice in this situation. For a nurse has a legal duty to warn of threatened suicide or harm to another following the requirements established by the *Tarasoff* court decision. In this case, that means that the nurse has a duty to warn the appropriate social service agency of the possible danger to the baby.

> I have been caring for a client with a history of manic depression who was just released from the hospital where she had been treated for congestive heart failure and cellulitis. She has bottles of pills everywhere in her apartment. Some bottles have only two or three pills; others are almost full. Old prescriptions for depression and expired medications for problems she no longer has are mixed in with her new prescriptions for her heart condition. There is no way to tell what she is actually taking. I did a mini-mental exam that convinced me she is severely cognitively impaired, though she insists that she can take care of herself. I don't think she will recognize that she's in trouble until it's too late. **Should a cognitively impaired client be the one to make the decision to live independently?**

Generally, treatment for mental illness can be mandated for competent clients who are judged dangerous to self or to others, and for clients who are incompetent, who can have treatment imposed if it is in their best interest. Some states also have a category known as "gravely disabled." Those who are classified as gravely disabled are unable to provide food, shelter, and clothing for themselves due to mental illness. The gravely disabled are deemed incompetent and therefore can be legally treated against their will.

Consequently, determining whether a client is competent is the crucial issue in many cases. To demonstrate their competence, adult clients must be capable of completing written forms outlining treatment and discharge plans (with help given to those with reading, sight, hearing, or speech impairment), and they must be able to repeat the treatment options, along with the benefits and burdens of each. Thus, a client's competency may be compromised if a client's cognitive impairment precludes the ability to acquire new information or weigh the advantages and disadvantages of treatment options, including treatment refusal.

Does this client's cognitive impairment render her incompetent? That depends on whether she can in fact explain her medications and the schedule and dosages she should take. If she cannot do that, the nurse should take the appropriate steps to begin the process of having her incompetence demonstrated so that treatment in her best interest can be mandated. This requires a probable cause hearing to determine whether she should be treated against her will. In the interim, the nurse should attempt to persuade her to destroy any old and expired medications, to diminish the risks in this situation. It is also important to document her concerns and her attempts to prevent harm to the client to establish her efforts to meet her professional duties to this client.

> Dual diagnoses clients are a challenge. If you were dealing with paranoid schizophrenics, you would know how to calm them down in a crisis situation. A paranoid schizophrenic with a cocaine habit is a different story. Their perception is much different. I have one client that I see weekly for court-ordered injections. Sometimes he frightens me, and I just want to leave. But I feel that I should be able to handle this. After all, I'm a professionally trained nurse. **Would I be justified in leaving a client's home if I am uncomfortable?**

Nurses must sometimes care for clients whose behavior is unpredictable and possibly dangerous. Although a nurse's primary commitment is to the client's health and well-being, nurses themselves have rights, including the right to work in a safe environment. Nurses are clearly within their rights if they take reasonable actions in order to protect themselves in such circumstances. This nurse is certainly justified in leaving a situation that makes her uncomfortable, as long as she makes the necessary arrangements to assure that the client receives the care he requires. For example, she could arrange to return with a police escort to administer his injection. She should also document this incident and inform her supervisor of her concern that this client may be dangerous. Of course, clients receiving court-mandated treatment are more likely to present these kinds of concerns.

ETHICAL CRITERIA

- A competent psychiatric client has the right to make free, deliberate, and informed decisions, including the right to refuse treatment.
- The psychiatric client has the right to truthful disclosure of information at an appropriate level.
- The psychiatric client has the right to privacy and confidentiality of mental health information.

PRACTICAL STRATEGIES

When a nurse is concerned about the psychiatric client's vulnerability to harm:

1. Take steps to minimize risks for the client.
2. Assess the need for intervention.
3. Support the right of competent clients to make decisions.
4. Monitor the situation for increasing dangers.

When others suggest withholding information from psychiatric clients:

1. Advocate for truthful disclosure.
2. Ensure that relevant material is presented to the client in an understandable manner.

When a client's family presents an obstacle to effective treatment:

1. Educate the family about the best treatment for the client.
2. Remind the family of the client's right to make treatment decisions.
3. Encourage collaborative or compromise decision making.
4. Report instances of suspected abuse.

When issues of whether to reveal confidential information arise:

1. Protect confidentiality as far as possible.
2. Disclose only what is necessary to protect the client's health and safety or the safety of others.
3. Review the legal requirements for nurses.

When clients are a danger to self or others:

1. Encourage voluntary commitment.
2. Contact appropriate authorities in cases of psychiatric emergency.
3. Act in accord with the duty to warn.
4. Document steps taken to address safety issues.

When psychiatric clients are nonadherent:

1. Attempt to determine the reasons for nonadherence.
2. Reinforce the need for the treatment.
3. Accommodate cultural beliefs and practices to the extent possible.
4. Seek mandatory treatment if necessary.

When psychiatric clients are suicidal:

1. Evaluate the client's need for hospitalization.
2. Emphasize the value of truthful discourse in order for accurate assessment and effective treatment of mental illness.

When clients suffering from psychiatric illness receive inadequate resources:

1. Act to safeguard the client.
2. Advocate for expanded access to address the client's needs.
3. Report incompetent professional care.

Chapter 10

CARING FOR CHILDREN

My client is a three-year-old child who has been comatose for three weeks. She has a brain tumor that basically takes up the whole brain. Because she is on Dilantin, she is getting home health care. The family wants to continue aggressive care, but I think that aggressive care is only prolonging the girl's suffering. **Who should make these decisions for dying children?**

General Issues

- **Who should make decisions for children?**
- **What special responsibilities do nurses have when their clients are children?**
- **When may treatment be withheld or withdrawn from a dying child?**

INTRODUCTION

Though nurses, technicians, and physicians provide the professional care children require when they are hospitalized, parents are expected to accept a substantial role when children are cared for in the home. If children are developmentally disabled, chronically ill, or seriously injured, this means that parents must learn to perform intricate tasks such as managing high-tech life-support systems. In addition, painful procedures that are performed by nurses and physicians in the hospital may be assigned to parents. They may be forced into the position of inflicting pain on their children by giving injections, or suctioning a trach, for example. Because parents want to spare their children any pain and unhappiness, their role in home health care may be profoundly upsetting. The parent-child relationship may be harmed as well, if children believe they can no longer trust their parents not to hurt them.

The dual roles of parent and caregiver consequently produce significant anxiety and distress. Adding to parents' distress is their sense that they have been forced to share control of their children's lives and well-being with outsiders who invade their family domain with intrusive schedules and procedures. Pervasive concerns about their other children and the ultimate prospects for the family in these circumstances exacerbate the stress on parents.

In response to these concerns, nurses strive to empower parents and families so that they have a sense of control and are able to cope with the tasks and burdens of caregiving. Nurses attempt to establish a collaborative nurse-family relationship, which is the key to the successful care of children in this setting. Given the vulnerability of children, though, it may be quite difficult for home health care nurses to relinquish control of their care to parents or families if they appear to be ill suited to these tasks. Their uneasiness about the care families provide or the decisions they make for their children are the source of particularly vexing issues for nurses who care for children.

MAKING DECISIONS FOR CHILDREN

When you're dealing with teen moms' their mothers and grandmothers tend to take over. I have a case right now where the baby had meningitis and is vent dependent; the mom is a seventeen-year-old girl who insisted she wanted to bring the baby home to care for him herself. Her mother called me to tell me that the girl doesn't take very good care of her baby. She had a doctor's appointment for the baby this week, but she made the decision that he didn't need to be seen. She skipped the appointment, so her mother wanted me to stop at the house to check on the baby. Then she said, "Don't tell my daughter I called." **Should this teenager be making decisions for this baby?**

Parents are recognized, morally and legally, as the natural decision makers for their children. They are assumed to know what is best for the child and to have the child's best interest at heart. Even in ordinary circumstances, though, this responsibility for making decisions for children can be overwhelming at first, especially if the parents are young and inexperienced. When a child is impaired or suffers from a chronic illness, the decisions required on their behalf become more complex and, subsequently, more daunting. Parents often lack the medical background to appreciate the full implications of the various medical options in cases like this. At the same time, they must cope with the emotional strain of adjusting to the reality of a baby who is medically fragile. Some would argue that parents should not even be asked to make decisions under these circumstances.

Though this mother would be recognized as the natural decision maker for her baby, it seems inappropriate to place the full responsibility for difficult decisions on a parent who is a teenager. This is a situation where a nurse should encourage this mother to seek the collaboration of others in making these decisions. Because the baby's grandmother has voiced her concerns about the baby, she may be willing to share some responsibility for the care of this infant. Through collaborative decision making, the teenager and her mother could seek to make decisions that address the realities of the care required for a vent-dependent infant.

If the teenage mom rejects any role for her own mother, the nurse should continue to emphasize the advantages of collaborative decision making. She could suggest that the girl seek someone else, for example, an aunt or a trusted older friend, who could talk to her and help her with the decisions she must make. The nurse should help them to identify the advantages and disadvantages of alternatives, answer any questions they have, and clarify their options to assist them in the decision-making process. The goal is to sustain the relationship between the teenager and her infant while ensuring that good decisions will be made for the well-being of the infant.

In addition, the nurse could seek additional services for this teen. She will need help, because caring for a high-tech infant at home ordinarily requires at least two adults who are trained and available, in addition to the home health care nurse. However, if the grandmother's concerns about the care the infant is receiving are substantiated and demonstrate that there is a serious threat to the well-being of the infant, the nurse should report this to the appropriate authorities.

I'm caring for a small child whose mother is a physical therapist. The physician ordered a medication for spasticity, two units to be given, four times a day.

Mom wants her son to have two-and-a-half units, and she wants me to give it. She should understand that I can't do that, but she is insistent. **Should parents be able to change the medication dosage that the physician ordered for their child?**

As the primary decision makers for their children, parents are allowed considerable discretion. Parents are allowed to make decisions for their children that are not the very best decisions possible, for example. They can even compromise the best interest of the child in order to accommodate what they see as the best interest of other members of the family. Moreover, when they must choose between treatment options, parents are allowed to choose or reject the recommendation of the health care team. Parents, for example, can refuse routine vaccinations for their children or use herbal remedies instead of other medicines to relieve cold symptoms.

However, the decisions that parents can make for their children are limited by law if the best interest of the child is at stake. For example, though competent adults could decide to stop treatment for themselves, parents could not simply decide to stop life-saving medical treatment for their child. Legally, the standard of best interest of a child is said to be violated if a parental decision puts the child at risk of serious, imminent, and irreversible harm. In such cases, parental decisions may be overruled. This is true even in cases where the parents are acting in what they believe is the child's best interest. Thus, a Jehovah's Witness may want to refuse a life-saving blood transfusion for an injured child based on religious tenets. Nevertheless, the courts will override both the right to exercise religious freedom and parental authority to make medical decisions for one's children in order to meet the state's duty under *parens patriae* to protect innocent third parties and speak for those who cannot speak for themselves.

Parents with medical knowledge, as is the case here, may assume that they know best what medications and what dosages their child should receive. The nurse should question them to determine whether there are changes in the child's condition or a concern about side effects or efficacy that is prompting the attempt to override the physician's order. This information should then be communicated to the physician so that he or she could decide whether to change the medications.

The nurse must administer the prescribed medication dosage, otherwise she could fail to meet the standard of care, and subsequently, could be legally vulnerable to charges of malpractice. She clearly cannot acquiesce to the mother's demands. When parents themselves alter a medication dosage or refuse to give it, a nurse must assess whether this is an example of medical neglect or abuse, which must be reported to the appropriate authorities.

> I am caring for a young girl whose mother has a significant anxiety disorder that prevents her from holding a job or going to school. She seems to be taking good care of her daughter, but sometimes her judgment is bizarre. Recently she has been insisting that her daughter wear heavy wool clothing even on the hottest days of summer. This is a huge issue for me. I'm concerned about her judgment, but if I report these concerns and she is hospitalized, she may lose custody of her daughter. She would be devastated by that, and her own health would probably deteriorate. **When should we say that a parent is no longer capable of making decisions for a child? Should the child's interests take precedence over the interests of her mother?**

The safety and welfare of a child client must always be the primary concern of nurses and others involved with the care of a child. If the competence of the parent or family caregiver comes into question, nurses do have a clear responsibility to report the situation. Even though the consequence of reporting may be loss of custody in a situation where a parent truly loves her child, decision making and care must be turned over to someone else if there is real risk to the child.

Nurses should exercise their responsibility to assess an individual's mental health and a possible need for hospitalization with great care, nonetheless. In this case the consequences of recommending hospitalization, for example, would be far-reaching and serious for both the child and her mother. To diminish the risks and the need for hospitalization, the nurse could attempt to discuss her concerns with the mother and suggest she contact her own physician for an evaluation of her health. She can continue to monitor the situation so that she can take more aggressive steps if the mother's judgment and behavior deteriorates.

There are a number of other ways in which safety concerns arise in pediatric home health care. Sometimes the home itself is unsafe for anyone. In other cases, the child has particular needs that cannot be met in the home, for example, when a child with respiratory problems lives in a house where temperature and dust cannot be properly controlled. Other family members can pose safety risks to an ill child if, for example, they smoke.

In all such cases, nurses should do everything they can to safeguard the child. They should intensify their efforts to educate the family, contact the physician, and report to child abuse teams when appropriate. Because state agencies seem slow or reluctant to take action, nurses need to become familiar with the criteria that will trigger a response and take care to phrase the appeal for help or intervention in terms that will result in action. Nurses must persevere in these efforts if their best assessment is that the child is unsafe in the home.

> I take care of an infant who has multiple neurological problems. The baby is extremely irritable. He cries when something touches him, he doesn't sleep, he can't stand to be held. In the beginning, even feeding the baby caused him to cry. The mother spends all her time trying to keep the baby content. They want to keep their baby at home, but the stress is evident. **Should I encourage them to have the baby placed in an institution?**

Though home health care is often the best care for a child, it is not always feasible. Even with the assistance of a professional nurse, parents may be unable to accomplish the mechanics of complex care. In addition, the responsibility and stress of caring for an impaired infant may overwhelm parents. In fact, the interests of the family may conflict with the interests of the infant, especially if the burdens of care substantially affect others in the family.

In their role as advocate for a client, nurses have the responsibility to act to ensure access to the level of care that best meets the needs of the client. However, home health care may not be substantially better care for this child, given the level of impairment. In many cases the child's level of awareness may be so limited that he will not notice the loss of daily contact with his parents. If that is the case, a nurse could encourage the parents to place the baby in an institution. She could lead the parents through a consideration of the costs and benefits of institutional care versus home health care, to help them reach a decision. This decision will most likely engender feelings of guilt and inadequacy in the parents, even if they believe it is a reasonable decision to make in these circumstances. The nurse can help them anticipate and deal with these negative feelings.

> I'm caring for a microcephalic girl who has a progressive orthopedic deformity. As she grows, her shoulders are moving forward and her body is curving inward. She is already having trouble breathing; she just had to have a bigger

trach implanted. Eventually she will smother if nothing more is done. Her mother wants to put her on a vent when it becomes necessary. I don't agree with her about this. **What should I do when I disagree with parents about what is best for their child?**

Decisions about their children are the legitimate right of competent parents, as long as the decisions do not constitute neglect or abuse. This child's mother has made her decision: though the ultimate outcome is unavoidable, she wants her child to be placed on a vent to assist her breathing, which will enable her to live longer. Being dependent on a ventilator as breathing becomes increasingly difficult, however, involves suffering that could otherwise be prevented. The nurse believes that makes it the wrong thing to do.

When nurses disagree with parents, the ethically appropriate response is to outline the reasons that lead to a different judgment about treatment. In this case, for example, the nurse knows that the use of a ventilator will cause some suffering for this child. She can provide information such as this that is relevant to the decisions parents must make. As an advocate for the child client, the nurse should advocate for what she believes to be in the best interest of the child. In the final analysis, though, the mother has the right to make the decision.

The principle that courts use in making decisions for children is the best interest standard: Which decision serves the best interest of the child? This is a deceptively simple-sounding principle, though, for well-meaning parties may have genuine disagreement about what the best interest is. When this happens, the substantive issue about best interest gives way to the procedural issue of who is the lawful decision maker. Parents have the legal right to make these decisions, but in a situation where the parents are in disagreement, it may be necessary to seek court intervention to determine what should be done.

One of the biggest issues for me is when a child is tested and found to be retarded. I have been caring for a young child, and that's the issue. The doctor hasn't told the parents what the diagnosis is. He isn't going to call it "retardation." He won't tell them "Your child is never going to do such and such." Now the child's mother is asking me questions: "What do you think is wrong?" **Should I tell her what I know?**

In order to make informed decisions about treatment, clients and surrogate decision makers need accurate and full disclosure of any relevant information. This is the reason that physicians are required to tell clients the truth about diagnoses, treatment options, side effects, and expected outcomes. Here the physician has failed in his duty to provide full disclosure. Though the diagnosis is one these parents will not want to hear, it is no kindness to delay their full understanding of their child's condition. Because he has not been forthcoming, the nurse has to contend with parents who expect her to provide this information. To answer the mother's immediate question, she can provide information about developmental stages, for example, and suggest sources of information that may respond to the mother's concerns. She should encourage the parents to ask their questions directly of the physician, and she should in turn advocate with the physician for a clearer and fuller explanation of the child's diagnosis.

Sometimes, despite the best efforts to inform them, parents seem to be in denial about the truth of their child's condition. Some parents believe that a miracle will happen and their child will be cured of his or her impairment. In such cases, there is not much that can be done other than to monitor the situation to be sure the child is receiving appropriate care.

SPECIAL RESPONSIBILITIES TO CHILD CLIENTS

With teen pregnancies you are sometimes dealing with certain social issues. Another nurse told me about a teenager who was pregnant, reportedly by the same boy who is the father of my client's baby. I wanted to say, "Check her for chlamydia" because I know the other girls he got pregnant. **What exactly would I be justified in revealing in this situation?**

Medical information must be kept confidential, even information about babies, children, and teenagers. Accordingly, information about the paternity of a client's child or about her health normally should not be shared with others, even other nurses, unless they are involved in her care. Confidentiality of such information can justifiably be breached only on the grounds that it is required by law or necessary to prevent harm. Granted that revealing the risk of clamydia to another nurse could be justified for that reason, the issue is how much should be revealed and, further, whether that information should be shared with the teenager's parents.

Because parents are the legitimate decision makers for their children, most feel they have the right to know everything about them. However, for purely pragmatic reasons, most states now grant minors over a certain age the right to confidential medical care concerning family planning, treatment of sexually transmitted diseases, and substance abuse. Otherwise, without the promise of confidentiality, minors are likely to go untreated, with disastrous consequences for themselves and public health. In this case, the nurse does not need to reveal the risk of chlamydia to the other nurse, because pregnant adolescents are routinely screened for sexually transmitted diseases. Thus, there is no justification for revealing any information at all about her own client to another nurse who is not involved in this client's care. The parents of the pregnant teenager should not be informed that she may be at risk of clamydia, either.

Parents and minors have the right to expect that information about the health of all family members will be kept confidential. The only exceptions would be the same as those for adults: Certain communicable diseases that pose a public health threat must be reported, along with suspicions of child abuse, and any injuries that suggest criminal battery, such as gunshot and stab wounds. Generally, information can only be released to schools, insurance companies, or others concerned with the care of the child, with the parents' consent.

> I have a case where the parents are completely stressed out. Their son was born with multiple physical and cognitive handicaps, and now that he's getting bigger, he's more difficult to care for. I'm beginning to suspect that the husband is hitting his wife. I observed two ugly bruises on her arm the last time I was there, but she denied that there was any violence. This last week they forgot to give his medications twice. My concern is that their child is not getting the care he needs under these circumstances. **What is my responsibility in this case?**

Nurses have special responsibilities when their client is a child who cannot advocate for himself. This may mean that they have to explore family relationships more aggressively than would be appropriate if the client were an articulate adult. When families are nonadherent, it is essential to inquire about their reasons for neglecting the medications and procedures that have been prescribed. Nonadherence may be the unintentional result of an increasingly stressful situation when parents carry the emotional and physical burden of caring for a seriously ill or handicapped child. If that is the case, nurses should increase their efforts to help parents find the resources available to them. Respite care is available in many communities, for example, to help parents in exactly these kinds of circumstances.

When parents are not carrying out the plan of care, this may be reportable as child neglect. There are two questions that can help a nurse to determine whether or not to report parents as neglectful: (1) Is the child at real risk? Are the parents making decisions that are genuinely harmful to the child? and (2) Would the child be better off staying with this family or being placed somewhere else? Given the difficulty of finding good placement for children with special needs, these questions should be considered carefully. The response of child protective agencies is often frustrating, because investigations are sometimes cursory and agencies appear to do nothing to address the concerns about child neglect. Moreover, such agencies are reluctant to separate children and parents, especially when alternative care for the child with special needs is difficult to arrange.

In general, one of the greatest problems parents face is learning about and gaining access to services. State, federal, and private practical help may be available, but complex bureaucracies and inadequate information about these programs are sometimes insurmountable obstacles for families to negotiate. For example, the Katie Beckett Waiver allows Medicaid funding for the home health care of children, regardless of parents' income or resources, if the child's disability is so severe as to require "institutional level care." But parents often need help in applying to this kind of program. Here nurses are an excellent resource for parents, because they can provide information and link families to the right agencies, or connect them with a social worker who can assist them.

It is well documented that the divorce rate of parents of children with chronic illness or psychological or developmental problems is much higher than average. Child abuse or domestic violence may also be a result of the frustration, stress, and disruption of the home that such families encounter. If evidence of child abuse or domestic violence exists, nurses should report this to the appropriate authorities.

What should the nurse in this case do, then? She should do what is possible to reduce the stress that may be a precipitating factor, observe the situation as carefully as she can, and report if the circumstances warrant it.

> My client is a four-year-old child who nearly drowned and is now vent depen-
> dent. She is very, very fragile. Her parents want her to have the experiences
> other children have. She is NPO, that is, she is not to have anything by mouth.
> Her parents have been feeding her anyway. I tried to explain to them that this
> is dangerous for her, but they think it is important that she be able to eat food
> like other children can. **Should I do anything else?**

Parents often want to provide their handicapped children with typical childhood experiences as far as it is possible. Many of these efforts
are beneficial to the child and family, but some are not. Though being
able to feed their child has important symbolic meaning for parents,
this is very risky for the child. Feeding a vent-dependent toddler by
mouth poses real danger of aspiration. The nurse should again attempt
to convince the parents of the dangers involved, and she must report
this to the child's physician. No nurse will agree to cooperate with such
medically dangerous behavior. In her absence, the child is vulnerable
to whatever the parents do in the privacy of their home.

> I am working with a family that is totally noncompliant, which is affecting the
> eight-year-old's health. This child is totally incontinent of stool and urine when
> she is angry. She is wearing pull-ups. I'm there to give enemas and monitor her
> diet. She lives with her grandmother, who has given up. She is not monitoring
> her medication; she expects the child to do that. There is no money for the
> proper high fiber diet, so she's not on the right diet. She needs a structured rou-
> tine, which she is not getting either. **How can I care for a child whose fam-
> ily refuses to cooperate?**

Children who are raised by family members with limited emotional or financial resources are particularly vulnerable clients when these
children have serious health problems. Their families may be unable
to consistently meet their responsibilities as caregivers or to supply
what the child needs in order to be healthy, the proper diet, for example. They may fail to provide the emotional support that enhances a
child's health. Community resources for caring for children like this
client, who have serious behavioral problems, unfortunately are
stretched thin. Consequently, many children who would benefit from
a structured environment, such as a facility with a staff of trained child
care workers and therapists, or temporary hospitalization in a child
psychiatric hospital, do not get it. Moreover, although medication can
be very effective in controlling many behavior problems, motivating

the child to stay on the medication is often a problem. Without the cooperation of their families, children often fail to get the proper medication.

In this case intervention is clearly needed. State agencies should be contacted, and a plea made for better arrangements for this child. Unless there is clear neglect or abuse, however, state authorities may not be able to act to change things.

> I am involved in caring for a two-month-old boy who is an anencephalic. Everything that is possible has been done to keep him alive. His parents are Muslim; they think he needs to be circumcised to go to heaven. His doctors are concerned that he might hemorrhage and refuse to do the procedure. The boy's parents are angry and extremely upset. **How can I be a successful advocate for this family?**

Even when their children are receiving home health care, the parents of infants with serious impairments often seem to be at the mercy of the medical system. They may believe the system prevents them from caring for their children as they see fit, especially when physicians refuse to perform a procedure or prescribe a medication a parent wants. On the other hand, parents should not be able to "order up" medical treatment; nurses and doctors are not mere technicians to carry out whatever procedures clients want. This means that the parents do not have the right to demand that the physicians carry out the circumcision in this case. The physicians can reasonably refuse, on the basis of their professional judgment that it poses an unacceptable risk of harm for this baby.

Because this infant will not survive long even with the best of care, the claim that circumcision poses an unacceptable risk is debatable. But the disagreement between parents and physicians goes deeper than that. This case presents a real clash of values: The view that physical survival is most important clashes with the view that the life of the spirit is more valuable. The tradition of Western medicine clearly favors physical well-being and makes little accommodation for parents with different values.

To advocate for this baby and his parents, the nurse could suggest finding a different physician who would be more willing to carry out the parents' wishes. She could also suggest that the parents consult their religious leaders to determine whether an exception to the requirement is possible in the specific circumstances of their infant. Some religions, for example, exempt hemophiliacs from being circumcised. Many religious leaders in the United States have found ways to accommodate their religious practices to the requirements of Western medicine.

> One of the cultural issues involves families that believe that everything is God's will. They don't believe in major medical interventions. "Whatever happens, happens." One case involves a baby who is very underweight for his age. He was born with neurological impairment associated with some retardation. He doesn't suck very well, so his nutrition is less than adequate. The doctors have suggested either a nasogastric tube or surgery to place a G-tube. They think they should try to have the baby removed from the home so they can treat him. **Should I support the parents or the doctors in this case?**

A religious philosophy that accepts all events as God's will is clearly at odds with a typical U.S. philosophy that God has given us the wisdom and technology to change things. From the perspective of the U.S. legal system, parents, doctors, and nurses are guilty of medical neglect if treatments are refused that could sustain or substantially improve the life of the child. Thus, unless treatment is clearly futile, parents can be required to accept it or lose custody of their child. Regardless of their own religious beliefs, then, parents must agree to the interventions Western medicine affords for their children.

There are some few exceptions, where courts have allowed minority groups to be exempted from laws about children. In general, the state has an interest in children and stands *in loco parentis*, in the place of parents, to assure their welfare. The state will not hesitate to intervene on behalf of the child in life-threatening situations. Consequently, even though the parents are opposed on religious grounds, the nurse should support the physicians and the decision to perform surgery in this case. She can try to help the parents understand that this surgery is legally required and attempt to help the family cope with the emotional burden of having medical procedures imposed on their child.

END OF LIFE DECISIONS

> I am caring for an infant who was born with very severe abnormalities; they basically sent him home from the hospital to die. His parents can't "let go."

They are waiting for a miracle. They insist that all his nurses agree to rush him to the emergency room for resuscitation if he arrests while they are there. **What is my responsibility? Should I agree to keep resuscitating him?**

For everyone involved, the decision to stop resuscitating an infant is wrenching. There is no clear-cut criterion outlining when it is ethically appropriate to withhold or withdraw a life-saving treatment. Generally accepted policy for newborns considers these things: treatment may be withdrawn if the infant is chronically and irreversibly comatose, treatment would merely prolong dying, treatment would not be effective in correcting all of the life-threatening conditions, treatment would be futile in terms of physical survival, or treatment would be virtually futile and inhumane. Considerations of the infant's quality of life, such as whether the infant is capable of any kind of meaningful relationship or whether the balance of painful sensations far outweighs any pleasures, may also be cited as justification for these decisions. All these criteria are controversial and open to interpretation.

If this infant is conscious and capable of suffering, withholding resuscitation and invasive treatment can be justified as a way to avoid pointless suffering. Also, his severe abnormalities could possibly justify such a decision on the basis of the infant's poor quality of life. However, the parents have the right to decide that they wish to continue aggressive treatment, despite these considerations.

Sometimes, as in this case, parents want to continue treatment, even when others believe it would be best to stop it. They interpret the slightest movement as an improvement or hold out with a strong conviction that a miracle will occur. This is difficult to counter, but continuing treatment of the infant in such cases amounts to using the child as a means to the parents' gratification and should not be encouraged. The nurse could bring her concerns to the agency's ethics advisory committee for their comments and suggestions about how to proceed in this case. A nurse may ask to be taken off a case where she disagrees with the treatment being given, as should be allowed by agency policies.

The client is a five-year-old child with muscular dystrophy. He is deteriorating, but his parents don't believe it. They want everything done for him. The nurses are in disagreement about this case; some of his nurses are trying to convince the parents "we can't stop now." I think they don't understand the dying process. I think we should "let him go in peace." **Should I go along with all this aggressive treatment?**

Decisions about stopping treatment for children with terminal illness may be even more difficult for parents than deciding for newborns, because the emotional attachment to the child is greater. Usually in such cases, decisions are based on an analysis of the costs of treatment in terms of suffering and lowered quality of life, measured against length of survival and enhanced quality of life. Nurses can advise, relying on past experience, but ultimately parents have to make the decision.

In some situations, a hospital-based nurse who has been caring for a critically ill child may "follow him home" and accept a position as a home health care nurse for the child. Parents might ask a nurse to become involved in this way, particularly when the nurse has cared for the child for several weeks in intensive care, for example. When this happens, there could be disagreements between the nurses from the "hospital culture" who are used to focusing on cure and aggressive treatment and other home health care nurses. Such disagreements should be discussed and resolved outside the home setting and without involving the parents. It may be necessary for the physician to meet with the parents to clarify what they want to have done. This is also a situation where a nurse would want to consult with her agency supervisor to determine how to handle this kind of disagreement. The agency's ethics advisory committee would also be a useful forum for discussing issues of professional disagreement.

> It's so tough when a child is dying, and he knows what's going on. I have a fifteen-year-old client who has relapsed after a lot of chemotherapy. They have run out of options, and he is going downhill pretty fast. His parents let him make all the decisions: whether to try a new experimental drug, whether to go back to the hospital or stay home. I admire their trust in him, but I think they may be giving him too much responsibility. **Should I say something to them about it?**

It is important to raise questions about the role of older children in making decisions about their own care. Adolescents can participate with surprising maturity even in life and death decisions. Though he is not legally an adult, this fifteen-year-old could certainly participate in the decisions that are being made. Whether he should be given complete responsibility is not as clear. It would be appropriate for the nurse to discuss this with his parents. She could also talk to the client to determine if he has questions or concerns that she can address. Most important, she can recommend that this family utilize collaborative decision making to reach these decisions. The client would still have a significant role, but he would benefit from the insights and advice of his parents, and he would be able to share the responsibility for these momentous choices.

Older children like this client should be consulted when a proposed treatment is experimental and is unlikely to be of direct benefit. Federal regulations say that children over age seven must give assent, and their parents must consent, for any non–therapeutic research. Children who wish to refuse experimental treatment may veto their participation in nontherapeutic research.

Children who have chronic illnesses tend to be very knowledgeable about their condition and their prognosis. They often will ask explicitly, "Am I going to die?" Nurses should discuss responses to this question with parents before the child has the opportunity to ask, and they should be prepared to respond tactfully but truthfully. They can attempt to assure the child that he will not be abandoned and he will not suffer. Finally, when children suffer from a long-term illness like cancer, they may indicate that they are tired of fighting the disease. The dying child's position should be taken seriously. Though the psychology of the dying child is complex, research shows that young children may know and understand more than adults realize, even if they do not talk about it. Helping parents to listen to their children is an important ethical task for nurses, especially in these circumstances.

This case also illustrates the fact that the general goal of facilitating health and healing may be replaced by the goal of palliative care and psychological support during the course of caring for a child with a terminal illness. Because hospice care for children is not always readily available, home health care nurses fill a vital role in responding to the special needs of families at such times. This allows the child and family to experience the comfort of remaining at home. The option to return to the hospital at the end should always be left open, however.

ETHICAL CRITERIA

- Children over the age of seven have the right to be informed about their treatment in age-appropriate language and asked to give assent to the treatment.
- Parents have the right to make decisions about medical treatment for their minor children and are entitled to give permission for beneficial treatment   even without a child's assent.
- Parents have the right to withhold or withdraw life-sustaining treatment from their children under certain circumstances.

PRACTICAL STRATEGIES

When concerns arise regarding the ability of parents to make decisions for their children:

1. Support the parents' efforts to act in the best interest of their children.
2. Educate the parents about available resources.
3. Contact the agency supervisor.
4. Assess the risk and act to safeguard the child.
5. Report medical abuse and neglect to the authorities.

When providing home health care becomes overwhelming for parents:

1. Advocate for access to care that best meets the needs of the client.
2. Contact the agency's social worker to advise parents about community support services.
3. Recommend institutional placement when deemed best for the child.

When the nurse disagrees with the family about what is in the child's best interest:

1. Contact the physician and agency supervisor.
2. Raise ethical concerns with the agency's ethics committee.

3. Educate parents about the consequences of their choices.
4. Advocate for the child.
5. Seek court intervention, if necessary.

When parents' cultural and religious values dictate nonstandard care for their children:

1. Assess whether there is a threat of serious harm.
2. Ensure that the parents understand the medical consequences and legal implications of their decisions.
3. Suggest a consultation with religious leaders, if relevant.
4. Report cases of abuse and neglect to the proper authorities.

When parents request futile or aggressive treatment for a dying child:

1. Explain the conditions under which it is legally permissible to withhold or withdraw life-sustaining treatment.
2. Support the parents' emotional needs and explain the role of palliative care.
3. Enlist the help of a social worker and identify community resources.
4. Consult the agency's ethics committee.

Chapter 11

SUMMARY AND CONCLUSION

Home health care nurses voice concerns that are compelling: How can nurses support a client's right to decide and also meet the responsibility to safeguard a client, if the client takes unwise risks? What is the responsibility of a nurse when family disagreements are affecting a client's health? How can nurses meet their commitment to client care if clients do not "follow orders"? Each chapter of this book begins with a case that illustrates one of these critical ethical concerns. This final, summary chapter reviews the general ethical issues raised by these cases and the decisions nurses must make. The discussions here will take a more analytic perspective than in earlier chapters, that is, the use of the various types of ethical reasoning outlined in Chapter 1 will be made explicit.

ETHICAL DECISION MAKING

I have a client who is dying at home. Her family has been wonderful with her. Her two sisters are taking care of her and they are with her all the time. She told me they pray together. She just seems so peaceful, even though her condition is deteriorating. Recently she obstructed, but she said she didn't want a colostomy. She didn't think her sisters could deal with it. **Should I support her decision to spare her family?**

Traditional methods of ethical decision making focus attention on two considerations: the moral and legal rights of individuals and the consequences of alternative courses of action. In effect, these methods address different aspects of a situation in which a decision must be made.

To reach a decision about this case, the nurse should first consider the moral and legal rights of the individuals involved. Given that this client is competent, she clearly has the right to make the decision to refuse a treatment option such as a colostomy. There are no rights of other individuals that must be weighed against the client's right to self–determination, in this particular context. Based on rights, then, the nurse would be justified in supporting the client's decision.

However, the consequences of the choice to refuse treatment could provide a basis for questioning the specific decision a client has made. This issue must be addressed when the decision will cause significant harm to other people. The impact of the client's decision here includes her own considerable discomfort and worsening health, but harmful consequences for the others involved appear to be minimal.

This ethical analysis will be incomplete unless an additional, important aspect of this case is considered, namely, the client's relationships. The client's concern for her sisters, together with her perception of her responsibilities to them, is relevant when the consequences of the client's decision are calculated. Moreover, this analysis must also take into consideration the facts of this particular context, where the care required after a colostomy will fall to the client's sisters. She is understandably concerned that they would find this a particularly difficult burden to bear. Thus an important consequence of her decision to refuse the colostomy is that her sisters will be spared the burden of providing that care. This supplies further justification for the client's decision.

When all these aspects of this particular situation have been considered, it is clear that the client's right to decide should be supported. Finally, the nurse should continue to advocate for any client's decision which is well-supported by ethical reasoning, even if she disagrees with the decision itself. Her professional and moral character is displayed in this commitment to client's rights even in that circumstance.

As this case illustrates, successful resolutions of complex ethical issues require going beyond traditional ethics to consider the significance of the context in which ethical issues arise, the relevance of the relationships clients have, and the character implications of possible courses of action.

CLIENTS' DECISIONS, NURSES' DILEMMAS

> One of my clients decided to live with his daughter so she could take care of
> him. He is supposed to be on oxygen all the time. His daughter doesn't want
> him on oxygen; she doesn't want her father to be sick. He needs a walker; his
> daughter tries to get him to walk without using the walker. I talked to her until
> I was blue in the face. I said, "You know he needs this." His daughter is in
> denial. She said, "He's getting better." He lets her tell him what to do. He wants
> to live with his daughter, but I think he is risking his health. **I have to let him
> make these decisions for himself, don't I?**

Generally, a competent individual's rights are the prevailing consideration in a situation. Competent adults have the right to self-determination, which includes the right to make decisions about treatment.
Even life-saving treatment can be rejected by a competent adult who
has made a voluntary, informed decision. Though this client has the
right to make these decisions, the nurse involved faces a moral conflict. She has a commitment to clients' moral and legal rights, but she
also has an ethical and professional responsibility for a client's health.
When clients exercise poor judgment, refuse necessary treatments, or
in other ways accept risks to their health and well-being, nurses who
reflect on the consequences will want to protect their clients from the
results of unwise decisions.

The traditional approaches to ethical decision making appear to
force a choice between respect for rights and consideration of consequences. But, as this kind of case illustrates, focusing exclusively on
either rights or consequences is an inadequate method for resolving
these issues. Attending only to the client's right to decide whatever he
chooses appears to mean that others have to stand by while he makes
decisions that will result in serious harm to himself. On the other hand,
focusing exclusively on the consequences of his decision may lead to
an illegitimate form of paternalism. Any interference with a competent
client's right to decide on the grounds that it is for his own good cannot be justified.

The nurse can begin to answer the question of how to advocate for
the client's rights and, at the same time, fulfill her commitment to the
client's health and safety, by thinking beyond rights and consequences. In this particular case, that means that she must consider the
client's relationship with his daughter. He has chosen to live with his
daughter and she in turn has accepted the responsibility for his care.

Clearly, this relationship is very important to the client, both emotionally and physically. The nurse should thus take into consideration the consequences for that relationship as she tries to determine what to do. Supporting the client's decision to continue living with his daughter will presumably enhance their relationship. If the nurse continues to address the daughter's denial, and tries to minimize the negative consequences, the client's relationship to his daughter will benefit, and the risks to his safety will diminish.

On the other hand, if she attempts to interfere with the client's decision out of concern for his health and safety, she will be forced to argue that the daughter's care harms her father. The possibly destructive consequences for the family relationship do not justify this response in this circumstance. Considering the effects on the client's relationships clarifies the decision: the nurse should support the client's decision to live with his daughter, despite the risks.

The nurse should also support the client's right to give informed consent for any treatments. Her continuing efforts to explain the risk of neglecting treatment are a way to ensure that the father's decisions are informed. In this way she acknowledges the client's decision to accept risks, while at the same time she is doing all she can to protect his safety and reduce the risks.

THE ROLE OF THE FAMILY

You need to have families involved in home health care, but it doesn't always work out well. Right now I am caring for a man who had a devastating stroke. His son moved him into his house to care for him. My client complained to me that his son is not bathing him often enough or feeding him regularly. Then he started to cry and said he didn't want to do anything to upset his son. He needs nursing care, but now his son wants to stop the home health care visits. **Should his son be the one to make these decisions?**

The client's son should not usurp his father's right to make decisions about care. This client ultimately has the right to make the decision to live with his son, despite the substandard care he provides, or to move out of his son's home, perhaps to a nursing home. The nurse can help the client think through what is right for him by spelling out the consequences, that is, the costs and benefits of these two choices. She can help him to think about what will happen to him if he agrees to stop the nursing visits. She can also guide him through a consideration of the consequences of a break with his son and the adjustment to life in a nursing home. In the end, if he decides that his family relationship is most important and that he will accept his son's decisions, that is his right.

Ideally, father and son would have utilized a collaborative or compromise decision making process to reach a decision that addresses the concerns of both of them. Though a nurse should advance a client's right to decide, in this particular context it is essential that she is also sensitive to the client's concern about his relationship with his son. The client wants to maintain a good relationship with his son, but he wants better care for himself, too. The nurse can respond to her concern about the son's neglect by attempting to re-educate him about his father's health care needs and the possible dangers of his own inattention to his father. At the same time she must be careful to protect the father's confidences and avoid antagonizing the son, because of the effect that could have on the family relationship.

Finally, if she believes the client's health and safety are endangered, she must report this situation to her supervisor and the appropriate agencies. Nevertheless, she should not pursue this matter with outside authorities unless there is some evidence of serious neglect or abuse.

SAFEGUARDING SECRETS, PROTECTING PRIVACY

One of my HIV patients is a forty-two-year-old male. He is so dysfunctional that he is not able to work. His HIV medications are paid for by a state subsidized AIDS program, which doesn't cover the antidepressants or pain medications he needs. He refuses to let me contact his parents for help. They don't know he is HIV-positive. **Should I talk to them anyway so he gets his medications?**

A client's right of self-determination is also the basis for the moral and legal requirement of confidentiality. Competent clients have the right to determine who has access to medical information and to decide the extent to which information can be revealed to others. From a legal perspective, confidentiality can only be breached when the law requires or authorizes disclosure of information. Disclosure is required in three situations: a subpoena has been issued for the information; disclosure is necessary to protect public health and welfare; and, disclosure is necessary to protect the client or an innocent third party from serious and imminent harm. In all other cases, the client must specifically give consent to have information shared.

In other words, the consequences cannot justify disclosing information about a client, except in the three kinds of situations identified above. Though the client's parents would probably want to help him obtain the medications he cannot afford, and the client would thus clearly benefit in that way, the nurse cannot decide to breach confidentiality on the basis of those benefits. The rules about confidentiality are not based on consequences, but on the right of an individual to have control over information about himself. Moreover, given the significance of family relationships, the client himself should be able to determine what his parents know about his illness. In that way he can retain some control over his family relationships. The nurse could attempt to persuade the client to reveal the nature of his illness to his parents, or she could seek other resources to help him pay for his medications, but that is as much as she can ethically do.

CLIENTS WHO DO NOT "FOLLOW ORDERS"

The client has intractable pain, congestive heart failure, hypertension and an anxiety disorder. Her husband says: "Whatever she wants, I do. If she wants to go to the ER, I take her." Last week they went to the Emergency Room on Thursday, Saturday, and Monday. If she doesn't like one ER, they stop at another ER on the way home. Sometimes it's for pain, sometimes it's diarrhea, sometimes it's constipation. She has medication she doesn't want to take, so they play around with her medications and then run to the ER. It's very frustrating. They're not managing her pain either. **What should I do?**

A nurse who is confronted with a situation where a client does not "follow orders" must determine whether this is in fact a competent treatment refusal, which is a client's right. If the client is exercising his right to refuse treatment, the nurse should respect that decision, under ordinary circumstances.

On the other hand, clients may be neglecting a physician's orders for several reasons: the treatment plan is too difficult to follow, medication side-effects are unpleasant, or some other goal or value is more important than adhering to the plan of care. For example, cultural practices and expectations sometimes conflict with the recommended treatments for a health problem. It is essential that nurses ascertain the reasons for a client's nonadherence so that they may address any problems with side-effects, difficulties adhering to a plan of care, or a client's depression. In each of these cases, nurses may appropriately focus their efforts on acceptable modifications to a plan in response to these concerns, and should discuss with the client's physician suggestions for changes which require a physician's orders. Also, nurses should act to assure that clients understand the nature of their illnesses and the consequences of nonadherence. The nurse's decision to respond in these ways is supported by attention to the client's moral and legal rights.

This may not be a sufficient response when a client's nonadherence raises serious concerns about the client's safety and health, as in the case above. With so many visits to the emergency room, something is clearly going wrong. The judgment of both the client and her husband is questionable, since they are apparently causing her additional health problems by modifying the medication dosages and schedules. In order to reach a decision about what to do in this particular case, the nurse should turn her attention to an evaluation of the consequences. It is clear that she should take some kind of action, since the negative consequences of the client's nonadherence are substantial.

First, she should redouble her efforts to teach the client and her husband about the effects of their nonadherence on pain management and the overall quality of life. She should contact the physician and advocate for a change in the medication orders, if she believes that will address the problems the client and his wife are apparently having with her care. If a nurse is concerned about self–neglect or the competence of a family caregiver, she should notify the appropriate supervisor and the physician promptly.

In some cases when clients are nonadherent, families and nurses must cope with the frustration of attempting to care for clients who resist their efforts to help them. Based on her rights as a professional nurse, this nurse could request to transfer care to another nurse, in accordance with agency policies and any applicable laws and regulations.

RESPECTING CULTURAL DIFFERENCES

> Since one of the local churches started sponsoring Haitian families, we some-
> times see clients who have unfamiliar ideas about diseases and medicines.
> Right now I have a client who is convinced someone put a curse on her
> because she suffered complications after she gave birth at home. She hasn't
> been taking her medications since she believes they won't do any good. She
> has a home remedy instead. **What should I do about her home remedy?**

Competent clients have the right to make decisions based upon
their own personal values and concerns, including cultural beliefs and
practices. This means that they have the right to make the decision to
reject Western medical practices in favor of cultural remedies, as long
as they have been fully informed about the consequences of that decision and the decision is voluntary.

The nurse should first make sure the client is well informed about
the nature of her illness and the prescribed treatment, in order to val-
idate her right to refuse treatment. Though the nurse is concerned
about the client's welfare, it would show a lack of respect for the
client's personal values simply to dismiss her cultural beliefs and
attempt to have her accept different values. Without disputing the
client's beliefs, the nurse may be able to persuade her to take the prescribed medication to relieve the symptoms she is suffering. This decision is supported by a focus on the rights of the individual client.

However, the nurse must also consider the consequences that may
follow from the client's insistence on the home remedy. It is imperative to determine what the home remedy contains, to decide if it is
harmful or would be harmful if taken together with the prescribed substance. If it is seriously harmful in itself, or if it interferes with a necessary and effective treatment, nurses have the obligation to ensure
that clients understand the consequences of maintaining the cultural
practice. The client has the right to continue her cultural practice, but
the nurse should not support this when the costs to the client outweigh
the benefits.

Finally, one of the reasons for respecting the client's beliefs is to support her relationship to her family and her own cultural community.
Though a nurse is justified in trying to persuade clients to follow prescribed treatment which is known to be effective, the nurse should
avoid alienating clients from their own community. However, cultural

practices which are illegal or pose risk of serious and imminent harm to others, especially a child or an incompetent person, should not be tolerated and must be reported.

FACING THE END OF LIFE

My client with end–stage cancer has finally decided he's through with all the chemotherapy. He told his sons he doesn't want to be resuscitated "if something happens." They're pretty upset about this. They don't understand why he doesn't want that. I don't know what's going to happen when he can't make his own decisions any more. **Should I intervene if his sons decide they will call the paramedics to resuscitate him?**

Competent clients can exercise their right to self-determination by completing an advance directive, such as a living will, which expresses their wishes about treatments to be provided when they are terminally ill and incompetent, or a durable power of attorney for health care, which names an agent to make health care decisions for them when they are incompetent. Comfort One bracelets, standard hospital bracelets with Allow Natural Death or Do Not Resuscitate printed on them, authorize emergency medical personnel to carry out an AND or DNR order in the home setting.

Consideration of the client's rights clarifies the decision that confronts the nurse in this situation. As a competent individual, this client has the right to refuse any life-saving measures. To promote his right to make that decision, the nurse should engage the client in a discussion of his wishes. If it is relevant, she can provide information about advance directives. She should emphasize that these documents must be executed while he is fully competent, before either the illness or pain medication puts his judgment in question. If he decides to complete an advance directive, he should be encouraged to provide copies to his sons, as well as his physician. He should discuss his wishes with his sons and make sure that they understand that this document is legally binding. In addition, he should arrange to obtain a Comfort One bracelet, which would allow paramedics to observe his wishes about resuscitation. If the client takes these steps, his sons should not be able to override his wishes about end of life treatment.

In any event, his sons would be wrong to attempt to impose resuscitation on him when he is no longer able to make the decision to reject treatment. The nurse should remind his sons that the client has made it clear that he wants no aggressive treatment in these circumstances. If they do attempt to override his wishes, the nurse should intervene to support the client's wish to reject resuscitation. She could present the advance directive or contact his physician for a DNR order, if that is necessary.

Further consideration of other aspects of the situation, most importantly, the client's relationship to his sons, also supports her involvement on behalf of the client. Encouraging a family discussion of these matters should foster a better relationship between father and sons. His sons would be able to voice their concerns and hopefully achieve an understanding of their father's reasons for refusing resuscitation.

The nurse should also discuss the services a hospice program could provide, since its philosophy is consistent with the client's wish to refuse life-saving treatment. Hospice staff have expertise in providing palliative care and can provide emotional support for the client and his sons.

If there is no advance directive, a surrogate decision maker should use any available information about the client's wishes regarding end of life treatment to make a decision on the basis of the substituted judgment standard. Absent an advance directive and reliable information about a client's wishes, a surrogate decision maker must use the best interest or "reasonable person" standard, choosing as a reasonable person would be expected to choose. Even without the information available about the client's wishes in this case, the reasonable person standard could support a decision to forego resuscitation.

NURSES' RESPONSIBILITIES, NURSES' RIGHTS

I'm working on a case now where the client's son is a doctor. He overrides the medication orders from her doctor, tells me to skip doses, and then when I don't do what he wants, he complains to the agency that I'm incompetent. His mother doesn't say anything. It's an impossible situation. **Would I be justified in refusing to care for this client?**

In both their professional role as nurses and in their personal lives as individuals with their own values and consciences, nurses can make justified claims on their own behalf. That is, nurses have rights, as well as responsibilities. Just as nurses have a professional responsibility to provide a caring relationship that facilitates the health and healing of their clients, they have the right to establish limits to the relationship with clients and families. For example, nurses are justified in refusing to meet demands that exceed their professional responsibilities. They are also justified in requesting to withdraw from a case where a family member is interfering with their ability to meet their responsibility to care for the client.

In addition to the client's right to make her own decisions, nurses' rights must also be considered in deciding what to do in the situation described earlier. When the client's son prevents the nurse from providing the medications ordered by the client's own doctor, his interference may make it difficult for the nurse to meet the standard of care. Her failure to satisfy the objective standard of care could subject this nurse to a charge of negligence or malpractice. For those reasons, the nurse has the right to object to his interference with the performance of her professional duties.

The consequences of allowing this situation to continue unchallenged also justify a decision to seek intervention from the client's physician or the home health care agency. The client may be harmed by the actions of her son when he insists, for example, that medication dosages be skipped. The nurse herself suffers from his unfair complaints of her incompetence, and she must also deal with the stress engendered when she is prevented from caring for the client in the way she believes is appropriate.

The nurse would thus be justified in requesting that she be allowed to transfer care to another nurse. In fact, she should suggest that the agency establish a contract with this client and family that would outline rights and responsibilities. Because the son's interference may make it difficult to meet the objective standard of care, the nurse must document carefully any of these incidents, and report them as necessary to the client's own physician and to her supervisor.

CLIENTS WITH MENTAL ILLNESS

It's the landlords who take care of so many of these clients who live alone. I have an elderly client with dementia who is hallucinating. Last week he thought the place was burning down. He was knocking on people's doors in the middle of the night and trying to drag them out of their apartments. His landlord called me to say, "Isn't this man a client of yours? You better do something. He shouldn't be living alone." **What rights does a client have in these circumstances?**

Competent clients who have been diagnosed with mental illnesses generally have the same rights as other clients. They have the right to make the significant decisions about their lives, including where they wish to live. Nonetheless, competent clients can have treatment mandated if they are deemed dangerous to self or others. In addition, some states classify clients as "gravely disabled" if they are unable to provide food, shelter, and clothing for themselves. Such clients are deemed incompetent and can be legally treated against their will.

At this time, the client in this case does not appear to be gravely disabled, or dangerous to self or others. Moreover, as a client with a mental illness, he is entitled to receive treatment that is effective in the least restrictive environment. For those reasons, he has the right to decide to continue living alone, in an apartment.

The nurse should monitor this situation as closely as she can, so that she can alert his physicians if he appears to need hospitalization for treatment of his mental illness. It should be noted that she cannot reveal confidential information about this client to his landlord. This would lead to loss of privacy for the client and could result in his eviction. There can be even more severe consequences to reporting this client's behavior to outside authorities. The client's condition might be a temporary condition that can be controlled with a change in medication, but someone may decide, on the basis of the landlord's description, that his behavior is grounds for involuntary commitment.

However, the special issues raised by clients with mental illnesses suggest that ethical also reasoning should focus on the consequences of the decisions made. The reason for this is that the consequences of a bad decision are likely to be serious and long lasting. The consequences of the client's dementia and hallucinations could be more serious the next time. The other tenants of this apartment building have the right to insist on measures to protect them from any possible harm from this client.

CARING FOR CHILDREN

My client is a three-year-old child who has been comatose for three weeks. She has a brain tumor that basically takes up the whole brain. Because she is on Dilantin, she is getting home health care. The family wants to continue aggressive care, but I think that aggressive care is only prolonging the girl's suffering. **Who should make these decisions for dying children?**

This case presents two separate issues about decisions for dying children. The first is the question of who has the legitimate authority to make these decisions. Moral and legal rights should be considered to resolve this issue. The right to make decisions for children who cannot decide for themselves is well established in practice and in law. Parents, whether biological or adoptive, are the designated decision makers for their children. If parents are not competent or if they have lost custody, a guardian is appointed by a court. Often grandparents or other family members are informally recognized as individuals who have the authority to make medical decisions for children. The question of decision-making authority becomes an issue only if there is evidence of abuse or neglect, or if life-saving medical treatment is refused for a child.

The second issue in this case is to determine what decisions are justified when children are dying. That issue is best answered by looking at consequences. Most often, a cost-benefit calculation will lead to a reasonable decision for a child with a terminal illness. There can, of course, be disagreement about consequences. Because cost-benefit analysis involves making predictions about the future, there is always some uncertainty and subsequently some disagreement. It is also true that people weigh the value of end results differently. Despite these complications, an evaluation of consequences is an appropriate method of ethical reasoning when someone must choose between alternative treatments for a dying child.

In this case, then, the nurse must defer to whatever decisions the parents make, unless their decisions raise issues about neglect or abuse. She can assist the parents in reaching decisions that reflect the important values they have, by offering to help them consider the consequences of pursuing aggressive treatment or withdrawing treatment for their child. In the final analysis, though, these decisions are difficult personal matters, and it is the parents who should have the ultimate authority to determine end of life care for their child.

Careful analysis of each of these cases demonstrates the usefulness of ethical decision making methods in resolving nurses' concerns. A consideration of the context, attention to relationships and to character are all indispensable to this analysis.

POSTSCRIPT

The voices of concern reported in these chapters result from the sincere desire nurses have to practice nursing with the highest level of professional responsibility and personal integrity. With changing social conditions and evolving nursing and medical practice, new questions continually emerge. The discussion offered here prepares nurses to reason well and to communicate with others effectively. The end of this book is only the beginning of the critical thinking and discussion that should be an on-going part of a nursing career. If these case studies motivate readers to continue thinking about ethics and this results in better client care, then the goals of this book will have been fulfilled.

LEGAL APPENDIX

Contents

Arato v. Avedon
Supreme Court of California, En Banc, 1993
S. Cal. 4th 1172, 23 Cal. Rptr. 2d 131, 858 P. 2d 589

The case against Dr. Avedon brought by Miklos Arato's family raises questions concerning the exact nature of informed consent, when information is material to a patient, the limits of therapeutic privilege, and whether it is ever morally and legally wrong for a physician to give a patient too much hope.

The widow and children of Miklos Arato, who died of pancreatic cancer, brought action against his treating physicians, claiming that they breached their duty to obtain informed consent for treatment by failing to disclose information regarding the life expectancy of pancreatic cancer patients. Miklos Arato was a successful electrical contractor and real estate developer when he was diagnosed with pancreatic cancer at the age of forty-two. Under the advice of his physicians, Arato undertook aggressive treatment for his cancer, including radical surgery, chemotherapy, and radiation.

Testimony indicated that Arato was informed by his physicians that pancreatic cancer is usually fatal, told about the unproven nature of the proposed treatment, and in light of that, the option of foregoing treatment altogether. Before his initial meeting with the team of oncologists, Arato had filled out a questionnaire with one hundred and fifty questions. Among them was a question about whether patients wanted to be told the truth or whether they wanted the physician to bear the burden for them. In spite of the fact that Arato made clear that he wanted to be told the truth about his condition, his physicians did not disclose to him the statistical life expectancy data for patients with pancreatic cancer.

The physicians claimed this information was not material. Material information consists of information that physicians know or should know would be regarded as significant by a reasonable person in the patient's position when deciding to accept or reject recommended medical procedure. Such information is needed to make informed decisions regarding proposed treatment. The patient's family claimed that had Arato known about the statistical morbidity associated with his disease, he would not have wasted his time undergoing treatment but instead would have spent his remaining months enjoying his family and arranging his business affairs. The false hope that led him to agree to treatment was a result of negligence on the part of the physicians, according to the Arato family.

Mr. Arato's treating physicians justified not disclosing statistical life expectancy data to their patient for various reasons. His surgeon testified that Mr. Arato had experienced a great deal of anxiety over his condition, to the extent that the surgeon was convinced that it would have been medically inappropriate to disclose specific mortality rates. Arato's chief oncologist, Dr. Melvin Avedon, contended along different lines that cancer patients "wanted to be told the truth, but did not want a cold shower." He argued that the direct and specific disclosure of extremely high mortality could deprive a patient of any hope of cure, which was medically inadvisable. Further, the physicians pointed to what little value predictive statistics were when applied to a particular patient with individualized symptoms, medical history, character traits, and other variables. They also testified that neither Mr. Arato nor his wife ever asked for information concerning his life expectancy in more than seventy visits over a period of a year.

The Supreme Court held that (1) physicians did not have a duty as a matter of law to disclose statistical life expectancy data; (2) evidence supported jury's finding that physicians reasonably disclosed information material to patient's decision; (3) physicians did not have duty to disclose information material to patient's nonmedical interests; (4) expert testimony regarding disclosure of statistical life expectancy data was admissible; and (5) erroneous jury instruction on physicians' duty was not reversible error. The court also held that the propriety of disclosing life expectancy information to a cancer patient depends on the standard of practice within the medical community.

In the Matter of Karen Quinlan, an Alleged Incompetent
Supreme Court of New Jersey, 70 N.J. 10, 355A 2d 647

The case of Karen Ann Quinlan was instrumental in establishing the right to refuse life– sustaining treatment under privacy rights against unwanted bodily intrusion. Since Karen was in a persistent vegetative state, this case was also significant in establishing the rights of guardians to discontinue extraordinary treatment used to prolong the life of an incompetent patient, without charges of homicide or wrongful death resulting.

On April 13, 1975, twenty-one-year-old Karen Ann Quinlan had been celebrating with friends at a birthday party when, after a few drinks, she began to pass out. Thinking Karen was drunk, her friends helped her to into bed so that she could "sleep it off." However, later that evening, when they went to check on her, Karen was found unconscious and no longer breathing. Two of her friends attempted mouth-to-mouth resuscitation and then rushed her to the hospital early in the morning on April 14th. Though she was found to have drugs and alcohol in her system, the levels were insufficient to have caused either a toxic or fatal reaction. Although the cause remained undetermined, Karen nevertheless had somehow suffered brain damage from oxygen deprivation, rendering her irreversibly comatose.

Karen's parents and sister and brother initially held out hope for a recovery. Karen seemed responsive to light and sounds at times. She would open and close her eyes, grimace, and make chewing motions. In spite of this, her condition rapidly deteriorated. Karen, who was five feet and two inches, dropped from one hundred and twenty pounds to seventy pounds and contracted into a fetal position. Her breathing was being done with the assistance of a respirator that had been placed in her throat after the doctors had performed a tracheotomy.

Karen's physicians at St. Claire's Hospital, Dr. Robert Morse and Dr. Arshad Javed, were in agreement that there was no reasonable hope of recovery from her coma. Further, even if she did make some physiological improvement, the overall quality of her life would remain the same. Three-and-a-half months after Karen was hospitalized, the family was reconciled to the fact that she would never regain consciousness. They also knew that she would not want to be kept alive under the circumstances. Yet, before making a decision to request discontinuing treatment, Joseph Quinlan, Karen's father, visited his parish priest. The priest, Father Thomas Trapasso, explained the Catholic church's position that there is no moral duty to use extraordinary means to keep a person alive. Now convinced that it was God's will that Karen be allowed to die, Joseph Quinlan went to the physicians and granted permission to have her removed from life support. On July 31st, the Quinlans provided written authorization to discontinue Karen's treatment and agreed not to hold the hospital liable for the outcome.

Although Dr. Morse assured the Quinlans that they were doing the right thing, the next morning he contacted them saying that he had changed his mind and could no longer go along with the removal of the respirator. One explanation for Dr. Morse's dramatic change of heart came from the hospital attorney who had notified the physicians that because Karen was legally an adult, Joseph and Julia Quinlan were no longer her legal guardians. In order for them to make the decision to refuse treatment on her behalf, they would need to seek legal guardianship in a court of law. Karen's father, therefore, went to court in an effort to be appointed guardian of the person and property of his daughter. If granted, guardianship would authorize him to discontinue all extraordinary medical procedures purportedly sustaining Karen's life. These measures, he asserted, presented no hope of her eventual recovery. In addition, there was no financial incentive for the family to request removal of treatment because Medicare was paying the $450 a day to keep Karen alive.

Quinlan's attorney, Paul Armstrong, appealed to three constitutional principles: (1) the right to privacy, (2) religious freedom, and (3) cruel and unusual punishment. The right to privacy, Armstrong claimed, includes the right against unwanted bodily intrusion. This allows patients and their guardians to refuse even life-sustaining treatment. The question to be addressed was whether the state's interests in the preservation of life and the prevention of suicide were compelling enough in this case to override the liberty and privacy interests against unwanted bodily intrusion.

Because Joseph Quinlan believed he was acting in accordance with the doctrines of his Catholic religion, Armstrong also argued on the grounds of religious freedom. To deny Quinlan the opportunity to act in accordance with these principles by having life support for Karen discontinued would violate Quinlan's first amendment right to religious freedom.

Finally, Armstrong argued that to keep Karen alive under the circumstances would violate her human dignity and constitute a form of cruel and unusual punishment in violation of the eighth amendment.

Judge Robert Muir of the New Jersey Superior Court ruled against Joseph Quinlan's petition on November 10, 1975. Muir found the state's interest in the preservation of human life overriding. Even though she was in a persistent vegetative state with no chance of ever regaining consciousness, because Karen had measurable brain activity, she could not be declared legally dead under the Harvard Brain Death Criteria. Because of that, Judge Muir considered the removal of treatment intended to end her life as an act of homicide and euthanasia. Though he did not question the good faith and motives of Mr. Quinlan, he believed Quinlan was too emotionally involved and distraught over Karen's condition to be appointed guardian.

Quinlan's attorney appealed Judge Muir's ruling to the New Jersey Supreme Court. Chief Justice Hughes described the significance of the case as follows:

> The matter is of transcendent importance, involving questions related to the definition and existence of death, the prolongation of life through artificial means developed by medical technology undreamed of in past generations of the practice of the healing arts; the impact of such durationally indeterminate and artificial life prolongation on the rights of the incompetent, her family and society in general; the bearing of constitutional right and the scope of judicial responsibility, as to the appropriate response of an equity court of justice to the extraordinary prayer for relief of the plaintiff.

Hughes ruled in favor of Mr. Quinlan, allowing him to assert a privacy right on behalf of his daughter. At the same time, he set aside any criminal liability that might result from removal of Karen from the respirator. He also suggested that the family consult with the St. Claire's Ethics Committee to determine whether there was agreement with the prognosis. Following a meeting with the Ethics Committee, Karen's physicians at St. Claire's weaned her off of the respirator. They did, however, express their intention to put her back on if there were signs of respiratory distress. They made clear that they did not want Karen to die under their care from the removal of the respirator, as they expected would happen. For this reason, the Quinlans had Karen moved to the Morris View Nursing Home. She remained there until her death on June 11, 1985.

Superintendent of Belchertown State School v. Saikewicz
370 N.E. 2d 417 (Mass. Supreme Court 1977)

The case of Joseph Saikewicz was significant in extending the right to refuse treatment to both competent and incompetent patients under certain circumstances.

Joseph Saikewicz was sixty-seven years old and severely retarded, with an I.Q. of ten and a mental age of two years and eight months, when he was diagnosed with acute myeloblastic leukemia. He had been institutionalized for the past fifty-three years and had been a resident of the Belchertown State School since 1928. Apart from the leukemia, Saikewicz was physically strong and in good general health. His severe retardation rendered him incapable of verbal communication, however, leading him to resort to grunts and gestures to express himself. One result was that Saikewicz was unable to respond to even simple questions regarding his medical condition, such as inquiries about whether he was experiencing pain. The only living relatives who could be located were two sisters who declined involvement in his case. Therefore, the superintendent of the school went to court requesting a guardian *ad litem* be appointed to make decisions on behalf of Saikewicz to determine whether he should undergo a course of chemotherapy. Given his age, stature, ability to participate in treatment and the stage of his illness, it was estimated that the treatment offered a 30 to 50 percent chance of remission, with an return of the disease in two to thirteen months. The disease will ultimately be fatal.

The guardian *ad litem* and Saikewicz's two attending physicians recommended against chemotherapy on the grounds that the burdens of treatment would outweigh the benefits. Although most patients with this diagnosis opt for chemotherapy, they accept the burdens with an understanding of the possible benefits. The hope, therefore, provides some measure of comfort. In the case of Saikewicz, he would experience the fear and physical discomfort of chemotherapy without being cognizant of the fact that it might be useful in prolonging his life. Moreover, the extension of his life was both uncertain and limited. Under the circumstances, Saikewicz's guardian was convinced that imposing treatment would be cruel.

There were three fundamental matters addressed by the Court in this case: (1) the nature of the right of any person, competent or incompetent, to refuse potentially life-sustaining treatment; (2) the legal standards that must be used to determine whether life-sustaining, though not life-saving, treatment should be administered to an incompetent individual; and (3) the procedures that are necessary to follow in arriving at the decision.

The Court ruled that the right to refuse life-sustaining treatment extends to both competent and incompetent individuals. The judge viewed the decision by the guardian to refuse treatment as consistent with the prevailing position in medical ethics that treatment should not be imposed when it offers no hope of recovery, where recovery refers not only to the ability to remain alive, but also to a life without intolerable suffering. He weighed the interests of Saikewicz in refusing treatment against the state's interests in: (1) the preservation of life; (2) the protection of the interests of innocent third parties; (3) the prevention of suicide; and (4) maintaining the ethical integrity of the medical profession. The judge allowed Saikewicz's guardian to refuse treatment on his behalf under an appeal to the "best interests" principle.

Cruzan v. Director, Missouri Dept. of Health
110 S. Ct. 2841, 1990.

In 1990, the U.S. Supreme Court for the first time made explicit reference to "a right to die" in its discussion of the now familiar case of Nancy Cruzan. In a 5-4 ruling, the Supreme Court recognized a strong constitutional basis for living wills and the designation of another person to act as a surrogate for medical decision making. The ruling was based on an appeal to liberty interests outlined in the fourteenth amendment to the Constitution. The Constitution also permits states, according to Judge Rehnquist in the majority opinion, to decide on the standard that must be met in determining the wishes of comatose patients.

Nancy Cruzan was twenty-four years old when she lost control of her car around midnight on an isolated, icy country road in Missouri on January 11, 1983. She was thrown thirty-five feet from the car and landed facedown in a water-filled ditch. A farmer noticed the headlights shining across his field and alerted the authorities. By the time paramedics were able to reach her, Cruzan's heart had stopped. The paramedics were able to restart her heart, but because she had been without oxygen for approximately fifteen minutes, Cruzan remained in a persistent vegetative state. For the next seven years, there was no change in Cruzan's condition. Because she was unable to swallow, she remained alive only with the help of feeding and hydration tubes. Unlike the case of Karen Ann Quinlan, however, which had become famous a decade and a half earlier, Cruzan did not need a ventilator. Thus, removal of the feeding tubes became the central issue in the Cruzan case.

In 1988, Judge Charles Teel of the Jasper County Circuit Court heard testimony from Nancy's parents, Louise and Joe Cruzan, and her sister, Christy, that Nancy said on many occasions she would not want to live under these circumstances. Judge Teel ruled in favor of their petition and granted the right to remove the feeding and hydration tubes based on the right to liberty of individuals to refuse death-prolonging treatment.

However, the Missouri Supreme Court in a 4-3 decision overrode the lower court's ruling. The reason was the state's living will statute that specifically forbade the withholding of food and water to hasten death. Judge Teel had argued in the lower court that Cruzan nevertheless retained the right to remove the surgically implanted tube used to administer food and water. But, because the Cruzans had not provided clear and convincing evidence that Nancy would have found the tube burdensome and intolerable, the judges found the state's interest in the preservation of life compelling in this case.

On June 25, 1990, the Supreme Court ruled that competent individuals retain a significant liberty interest in remaining free from unwanted bodily intrusion. In this case, our use of technology led to a sustaining of life that actually interfered with individual liberty. Addressing the issue of incompetent patients, the Court set a standard for clear and convincing evidence regarding patients' wishes concerning treatment refusal under the circumstances. Therefore, the Supreme Court refused to reject the legal standard set by the state of Missouri, which would have overturned the appellate court's decision. Nevertheless, they left the door open for the Cruzans to go back to the Circuit Court and provide the clear and convincing evidence required to demonstrate that Nancy would have found the feeding tubes intolerable. On December 14, 1990, Judge Teel accepted the evidence offered by family and friends of Nancy Cruzan and ordered the feeding and hydration tubes removed. Cruzan died twelve days after the removal of the tubes on December 26, 1990.

In the same year that the Supreme Court made a decision in the Cruzan case, federal legislation was passed aimed at protecting the rights of patients in such medical crises. The Patient Self-Determination Act of 1990 mandates that each patient be informed of the right to exercise treatment preferences, including preferences concerning life-sustaining measures.

The Case of Joyce Brown versus Mayor Ed Koch

This case illustrates some of the challenges associated with assessing dangerousness and outlines the various conditions that must be met under governmental powers to involuntarily commit those who suffer from mental illness.

Joyce Brown, known to the public as "Billie Boggs," became famous for being at the center of a legal battle to determine the rights of the mentally ill against involuntary commitment. Boggs was a forty year old who survived on the streets of New York City. To the dismay of those she encountered in the affluent Manhattan neighborhood whose streets she wandered, Boggs engaged in a range of bizarre behaviors, some of which were violent. She would expose herself, speak in rhymes that were sexual in content, and tear up money and urinate on it. She was often filthy and smelled of urine and excrement. Mayor Koch's administration had implemented a program known as "Project Help" to evaluate homeless mentally ill individuals for potential psychiatric treatment. Boggs' actions and lifestyle prompted the concern of emergency psychiatric services personnel, who diagnosed her as suffering from serious mental illness. Social service employees at New York City Health and Hospital Corporation sought to have Boggs involuntarily committed for treatment. This action was vehemently opposed by the New York Civil Liberties Union, who argued that Boggs was in her current plight due to homelessness rather than significant mental illness. The Civil Liberties Union contended that forced evaluation leading to involuntary commitment would surely violate the rights of the mentally ill. On October 28, 1987, Boggs was forcibly removed from the street and brought to the emergency room at Bellevue Hospital. She was treated and moved to a locked psychiatric ward. She called the ACLU from there, and their lawyers agreed to represent her on the condition that they could use her story to publicize the plight of the homeless.

When Boggs's story was broadcast on television, three women came forward and identified her as their sister. They told the story of a bright, happy, attractive child from New Jersey, who was a successful student and business school graduate. She worked for both Bell Laboratories and the New Jersey Human Rights Commission before becoming dependent on heroin and cocaine. During this same time, she was diagnosed as psychotic and involuntarily committed by her sisters for treatment. When she was released two weeks later, she went to the east side of Manhattan and began living on the streets.

Traditionally, two governmental powers have been applied to justify involuntary treatment of individuals with significant mental illness. The first is the police power that is invoked by governments to protect citizens from the harmful actions of others. The second is the power of *parens patriae*. The state is parent to its citizens and as such is responsible for the care of those who are unable to care for themselves, including the mentally disabled.

In meeting its duties toward citizens, the state uses both criminal and civil commitment to promote safety and welfare. Further, civil commitment of an individual who suffers from mental illness has been justified by appeal to both powers to protect the individual from harming herself and to prevent harm from coming to others. Thus, there were two sections of New York's Mental Hygiene Law that could have been applied. Under the *parens patriae* statute, the state needed to demonstrate that Boggs suffered from a mental illness and that treatment in a hospital was appropriate, her welfare was impaired, and she was incapable of understanding her need for treatment.

However, in Boggs's case, a more stringent standard was agreed upon by the court. Beyond meeting the conditions necessary under *parens patriae*, the state required the H.H.C. to demonstrate the likelihood of serious harm to self or others. The proof of dangerousness was necessary to invoke the use of police powers to achieve civil commitment.

Conflicting testimony of experts provided little guidance for the judge, Robert Lippman, who ultimately relied on his own assessment of Boggs and ordered her released. A five-judge appeals court found Lippman in error (3-2) and accepted H.H.C.'s proof of dangerousness. Yet, because Boggs was entitled to refuse psychotropic medication, she was released from the hospital on the grounds that without treatment, it would serve no purpose.

Boggs became a celebrity for a while, accepting job offers and television appearances, and speaking at law schools on behalf of the homeless. She ended up back on the streets, however, all the while maintaining that she was not insane, simply homeless.

Warthen v. Toms River Community Memorial Hospital
101 N.J. 255, 501 A.2d 926 N.J., 1985

A nurse's primary responsibility as a patient advocate will, at times, lead to conflicts between a nurse's ethical duty to her patients and the legal duty she has to her employer and the physician. Such conflicts pose the potential for serious professional risk. A nurse who is ordered by a physician to perform acts she considers unethical or which are illegal or not in the best interest of the patient must decide personally and professionally how much to risk for the sake of practicing nursing according to the standards she has set for herself. Conflicting rulings in the courts provide little guidance for nurses in assessing these risks. Nevertheless, there are cases that provide an outline of how the courts have dealt with employer's efforts to limit the nurse's role as a patient advocate.

One of the mostly highly publicized cases was *Warthen v. Toms River Community Memorial Hospital.* Corrine Warthen worked as a nurse specialist in kidney dialysis at Toms River Community Memorial Hospital in New Jersey. She was assigned to dialyze a terminally ill double-amputee patient who was in renal failure. On two prior occasions, Warthen was forced to halt the procedure because the patient suffered both severe internal hemorrhaging and cardiac arrest. Warthen was opposed to further dialysis for this patient on moral grounds. In accordance with the ANA code, she notified her supervisor in a timely manner of her objections to performing a procedure that she opposed morally and professionally. Warthen was convinced that further treatment was not in the patient's best interest. She attempted to appeal to the ANA code to justify her refusal of care on the grounds that the code mandates respect for human dignity. Warthen believed the patient's human dignity was violated by continued attempts at dialysis. When Warthen was fired, she used a public policy defense to make a claim of wrongful discharge.

According to the employment-at-will doctrine, employment can be terminated by either party without there being a cause for legal action. Warthen was seeking an exception to this doctrine on the grounds that when she failed to follow orders, she was acting justifiably in accordance with her professional code. There was legal precedent for such an appeal. In *Pierce v. Ortho Pharmaceutical Corp.*, the court recognized that professional employees owe a special duty to abide by the recognized codes of ethics within their professions, as well as state and federal laws. However, the court held that an employee has a cause for action for wrongful discharge only when the discharge is contrary to a "clear mandate" of public policy. The burden of proof is on the employee to identify the expression of public policy in the code. The court found against Warthen because her acts, although done for the sake of the patient, could not be shown to benefit the public to such an extent that they would constitute a public policy exception to the employment-at-will doctrine. Public policy exceptions are based on the premise that allowing the employer to fire the employee under the circumstances would go against the public good and should therefore be prohibited. New Jersey's Supreme Court had also just passed a law upholding patients' rights to expect that medical treatment will not be terminated against their will. The court was concerned about potential conflicts if nurses were allowed to withdraw from cases for moral reasons. Patients' rights, the court insisted, must remain paramount.

The implications of this case for the home health care nurse are far-reaching. Like Warthen, a nurse may be acting from conscience out of concern for patient welfare and safety. Further, because of the importance of the nurse-patient relationship, a nurse's role as advocate may legitimately fall under the purview of public welfare. Yet, this is not sufficient to provide the clear mandate sought by the courts. In the absence of state statutes and case law supporting nurses' acts of refusal, the nurse is left without legal protection from dismissal by the agency and perhaps even loss of her license.

Lampe v. Presbyterian Medical Center
41 Colo. App. 465 P2d. 513, 1978

> *Nurses' acts of advocacy are not without their risks, however. In the case of* Lampe v. Presbyterian Medical Center, *the plaintiff, who was the head nurse of an intensive care unit, brought suit against her employer for retaliatory discharge on the grounds that her termination violated a mandate of the Colorado Nurse Practice Act. This case sheds light on the status of professional codes for nurses in courts of law.*

The plaintiff, Lampe, was responsible for staffing the intensive care unit at the Presbyterian Medical Center. When she was ordered to reduce overtime expenditures, she refused to do so out of fear of jeopardizing the health and safety of her patients. Lampe was subsequently fired for her unwillingness "to fulfill the requirements of her job description."

Lampe appealed to her state's Nurse Practice Acts, which required a nurse to act in manner consistent with the health and safety of her patients. According to Lampe, if she had followed orders to reduce the overtime of her staff, she would have violated the statute under which she was licensed. However, the court refused to recognize the Nurse Practice Acts as sufficient to "modify the contractual relationships between hospitals and their employees in such situations."

The dilemma faced by Lampe is a familiar one for home health care nurses who practice in a time of managed care. Home health care nurses are often torn between an agency's mandate to visit a certain number of patients within a short period of time and the needs of patients who require lengthier, more frequent, or continued visits.

Tuma v. Board of Nursing
100 Idaho 74, 593 P. 2d 711, 1979

The Nurse Practice Acts have been used by both sides in claims of wrongful discharge by nurses acting in their roles as patient advocates. This case centers on the limits of that role and the issue of whether providing a patient with requested information about alternative treatments for cancer constitutes unprofessional conduct in violation of the Nurse Practice Acts.

In *Tuma v. Board of Nursing,* Tuma, a clinical nursing instructor, requested the assignment of administering chemotherapy to a patient with leukemia. Tuma was concerned about addressing the needs of dying patients. This particular patient reportedly pleaded with Tuma to return in the evening, after the treatment, to discuss an alternative to the chemotherapy. Tuma agreed and discussed the possibility of laetrile and dietary therapy with the patient. Unfortunately, the patient died two weeks later as a result of experiencing serious adverse side effects from the chemotherapy.

Although no one contended at the trial that Tuma's actions in any way caused harm to the patient, hospital personnel contacted the Idaho State Board of Nursing and complained that Tuma had interfered with the physician-patient relationship. A hearing officer concluded that Tuma's discussion of treatment alternatives with her patient did in fact constitute unprofessional conduct in violation of the

Idaho Nurse Practice Act. The Board of Nursing upheld the hearing officer's decision and suspended Tuma's license for six months.

Tuma won her case on appeal. The Idaho Supreme Court cited the Minimum Standards, Rules, and Regulations put forth by the Idaho Board of Nursing, which require nurses to promote patient education based on the individual's health needs. Tuma's actions were consistent with this mandate. Therefore, the Court held that the Board of Nursing violated Tuma's rights by authorizing the suspension of her license in the absence of a specific statutory definition of what constitutes unprofessional conduct.Home health care nurses, in their role as patient advocate, should be familiar with the laws in their state covering nursing practice and the extent and limitations of the protections provided by state statute and other public policy mandates. The Nurse Practice Acts are often too vague and broad to provide clear guidance to the courts. As a consequence, nurses who believe they are doing what is required of them as a nurse can be subject to disciplinary action, including dismissal, without any recourse in the courts.

Tarasoff v. Board of Regents of University of California 529 P 2d 553 CA, 1976.

Tarasoff v. Board of Regents of University of California has had a substantial impact in relation to the law surrounding misfeasance—the duty to prevent harm. The resulting ruling from this case was that the duty to confidentiality must be breached when there is a threat of serious imminent harm to an innocent third party. While psychiatrists at the time of the decision were concerned about its effects on the willingness of patients to disclose information necessary for their treatment, their fears have proved unwarranted in the years following this case.

Prosenjit Poddar became obsessed with nineteen-year-old Tatiana Tarasoff. After she made clear to Poddar that she had no interest in a relationship with him, he sought psychiatric care from a staff psychologist at the University of California's student counseling center. Poddar confessed homicidal thoughts to the psychologist, who immediately contacted campus security. The psychotherapist expressed concern regarding Poddar's dangerousness and requested involuntary commitment of Poddar for observation and treatment. Upon questioning by the police, Poddar promised to stay away from Tarasoff and convinced them that he posed no real danger to her or himself. He then discontinued counseling and, two months later, killed Tarasoff. Her parents successfully sued the university for both failure to detain Poddar and failure to warn their daughter. The court thus upheld a duty on the part of psychiatrists to warn innocent third parties of threats directed at them by psychiatric patients.

In re Baby K.
16 F. 3d. 590; 1994 U.S. Court of Appeals

The case of Baby K. raises important questions regarding what constitutes futile treatment and who should be allowed to make the determination. Baby K. was born with anencephaly. The life expectancy for infants born with just a brain stem ranges from a few hours to a few weeks. Death usually results from respiratory failure due to the inability of the brain stem to regulate breathing. In spite of the fact that even if she were to survive, her daughter would never have the capacity for thought, Baby K.'s mother sought aggressive treatment against the wishes of health care providers.

Baby K. was born in Fairfax Hospital in Falls Church, Virginia, in 1993. Suffering from anencephaly, her mother was told that the standard treatment for babies born with this condition was to be kept comfortable until their organ systems fail, which most often occurs within a few weeks. Baby K.'s mother, who had deeply held Christian beliefs that all life should be protected, wanted everything medically possible done for her child.

Baby K. was cared for in a nursing home. At sixteen months, she required two hospitalizations for respiratory problems. Following her second hospitalization, Fairfax Hospital went to court seeking a ruling that would allow them to refuse what the doctors considered to be futile treatment for Baby K., given that her medical condition would not improve as a result. In spite of a hospital ethics committee ruling in support of discontinuation of aggressive treatment, the district court found in favor of Baby K.'s mother.

The hospital, along with Baby K.'s father, appealed to the U.S. Court of Appeals. This court applied the standards of the Federal Emergency Medical Treatment Act, which prohibits the abandonment of individuals in medical emergencies. Even though Baby K.'s treatment exceeded the prevailing standards of medical care, the court ruled that there were no exceptions passed by Congress that would preclude treatment just because it might not be expected to provide a medical benefit. Thus, Baby K.'s mother won the right to have her treated against the wishes of physicians who considered the treatment futile.

GLOSSARY

Abandonment: The improper termination of the relationship between a professional caregiver and patient.

Advance directive: A legal document through which an individual may provide directions or wishes as to medical care. It is used when the person is unable to make or communicate decisions about medical treatment and prepared before any condition or circumstance occurs that renders the patient incapable of actively making a decision regarding medical care.

Assent: A weakened form of consent given by minors.

Assisted suicide: Assisting a patient by providing the means for the individual to take his or her own life.

Attorney-in-fact for health care decisions: A person named by the patient in a document called a durable power of attorney, to make decisions other than the withdrawal of life support systems. An attorney-in-fact may make decisions about any aspect of medical care, except (1) withdrawal of life support systems, (2) withdrawal of food and fluids, and (3) medical treatment designed solely to maintain physical comfort.

Authenticity: In cases of substituted judgment, the concept of authenticity requires that decisions be made for clients that are consistent with their values and the way they lived their lives.

Autonomy: The right to determine what happens to one's own body based on one's values. Autonomous decisions are free, deliberate, informed, and lead to self-governed action.

Battery: The unlawful touching of another person without the individual's permission. Battery occurs in the context of medical care when the treatment exceeds what the patient has consented to, constituting technical battery for which the patient may seek redress.

Beneficence: Doing or promoting good and well-being.

Best interest standard: A decision by a surrogate decision maker based on what would be in the client's best interest.

Breach: Failure to meet a legal duty either by acting or failing to act.

Code of ethics: Codes put forward by professional organizations, outlining responsibilities in the context of professional-client relationships.

Collaborative decision making: The process whereby clients retain their central role in making final decisions for themselves but reach their decisions after consultation with their families or others.

Comfort One: A program enacted to allow patients to signal treatment refusal by wearing bracelets in cases where the individual becomes incapacitated and is unable to communicate end-of-life wishes.

Compromise decision making: A decision-making process in which competent clients who have clear ideas about what they want are willing to shape their decisions in response to the wishes of others through a process of negotiation and compromise.

Competence: The mental ability to make judgments based on a certain level of rationality.

Compliance: A client or family's adherence with a plan of care prescribed by professional caregivers.

Consequentialist ethical theories: For consequentialists, the rightness and wrongness of acts is determined solely by the consequences of the acts. Right acts produce the best possible consequences for everyone involved than any alternative act.

Conservator of the person: A conservator is someone appointed by the Probate Court when the Court finds that a person is incapable of making decisions about his or her healthcare. This person has the power to give consent for medical care, treatment, and services provided to the incapable person.

Confidentiality: Informational privacy between health care professionals and their clients.

Damages: Monetary compensation awarded by the courts for injury sustained to one's body or property due to negligence on the part of another party who owed a duty.

DNR code: A do not resuscitate code or "no code" indicates not to resuscitate the patient in the event of cardiac arrest.

Doctrine of double effect: The Christian doctrine according to which acts having both good and bad consequences are morally permissible. Such acts must be good or neutral in and of themselves. The good consequences and not the bad must be intended. The bad consequence cannot be used as a means to bring about the good consequences. Finally, the good consequences that are brought about must be proportionate to or greater than the bad consequences.

Durable power of attorney: A type of advance directive in which a person is designated as a decision maker for medical questions that arise if the client becomes incapacitated.

Emancipated minor: Someone under the age of majority who lives independent of his or her parents. An emancipated minor can legally consent to treatment and is responsible for his or her own debts.

Euthanasia: The intentional taking of another's life or the refraining from acts that could prolong another's life out of considerations of mercy. Active euthanasia involves the intentional taking of another's life, whereas passive euthanasia is the withholding of treatment that could prolong a person's life.

Extraordinary means: Means used to prolong a patient's life where the physical, emotional, and financial burdens outweigh the benefits of the treatment.

Health care agent: A person authorized in writing by the patient to convey wishes concerning the withholding or withdrawal of life support systems. The agent does not become involved in any other treatment decisions.

Heroic measures: Extraordinary means used to prolong a person's life.

Individualistic decision making: Decision-making process where clients think through the issues independently and reach a unilateral decision.

Informed consent: A patient's permission to provide medical care following disclosure of relevant information, requiring the capacity on the part of the patient to make a competent decision, an understanding of the information presented, and the absence of coercion.

Incompetence: The physical or mental incapacity to carry out one's affairs. Incompetent patients cannot enter into contracts.

Life support system: A form of treatment that delays the time of death or maintains the patient in a state of permanent unconsciousness. These include among others: respirators and dialysis, cardiopulmonary resuscitation, artificial nutrition and hydration, and antibiotics in certain circumstances.

Living Will: A document that states whether a person wishes to have administered life-sustaining procedures or treatments in the event of a terminal condition or being in a state of permanent unconsciousness. A Living Will goes into effect only when (1) the individual is unable to make or communicate decisions about health care and (2) is in a terminal condition or permanently unconscious.

Mature minor doctrine: Legal status given under common law for minors to consent to care.

BIBLIOGRAPHY

Books

Andrews, Margaret M. and Joyceen S. Boyle, (Eds.): *Transcultural Concepts in Nursing Care*, 2nd edition. Philadelphia, J. Lippencott Company, 1995.

Arras, John D., Porterfield, H. William, and Porterfield, Linda Obenauf, (Eds.): *Bringing the Hospital Home: Ethical and Social Implications of High-Tech Home Care.* Baltimore and London, Johns Hopkins University, 1995.

Benjamin, Martin, and Curtis, Joy: *Ethics in Nursing.* New York, Oxford University, 1991.

Bishop, Anne H., and Scudder, Jr., John R., (Eds.): *Caring, Curing, Coping: Nurse, Physician, Patient Relationship.* Birmingham, University of Alabama, 1985.

_____: *Nursing Ethics: Therapeutic Caring Presence.* Belmont, Wadsworth, 1996.

Clemen-Stone, Susan, McGuire, Sandra L., and Eigsti, Diane Gerber, with contributions by Brook, Ella M., Eds. *5th Comprehensive Community Health Nursing. Family, Aggregate, and Community Practice.* St. Louis, Mosby, 1998.

Davis, Anne J., Aroskar, Mila A., Liaschenko, Joan, and Drought, Theresa S., (Eds.): *Ethical Dilemmas and Nursing Practice.* Upper Saddle River, Prentice Hall, 1996.

Galanti, Geri-Ann: *Caring for Patients from Different Cultures: Case Studies from American Hospitals.* Philadelphia, University of Pennsylvania, 1997.

Gubrium, Jaber F., and Sankar, K. Pal : *The Home Care Experience.* Thousand Oaks, Sage, 1990.

Haddad, Amy Marie, and Kapp, Marshall B.: *Ethical and Legal Issues in Home Care: Case Studies and Analyses.* Norwalk, Appleton and Lange, 1991.

JCAHO: *Framework for Improving Performance: A Guide for Home Care and Hospice Organizations.* Oakbrook Terrace, 1995.

Henderson, Virginia: *The Nature of Nursing.* New York, MacMillan, 1966.

Kane, Rosalie A., and Caplan, Arthur L.: *Everyday Ethics: Resolving Dilemmas in Nursing Home Life.* New York, Springer, 1989.

Keltner, Norman L., Schwecke, Lee Hilyard, Bostrom, Carol E.: *Psychiatric Nursing,* 3rd edition. St. Louis, Mosby, 1995.

Marrelli, Tina M.: *Hospice and Palliative Care Handbook. Quality, Compliance, and Reimbursement.* St. Louis, Mosby, 1999.

Moody, Harry R.: *Ethics in an Aging Society.* Baltimore, John Hopkins University, 1992.

Nelson, James Lindemann, and Nelson, Hilde Lindemann: *The Patient in the Family: An Ethics of Medicine and Families.* New York, Routledge, 1995.

Potter, Patricia A., and Perry, Anne Griffin: *Fundamentals of Nursing* , 5th ed. St. Louis, Mosby, 2001.

Rice, Robin. *Home Health Nursing Practice Concepts and Application,* 2nd ed. St. Louis, Mosby, 1996.

Robbins, Dennis A.: *Ethical and Legal Issues in Home Health and Long Term Care: Challenges and Solutions.* Gaithersburg, Aspen, 1996.

Stanhope, Marcia, and Lancaster, Jeannette: *Community Health Nursing: Process and Practice for Promoting Health,* 3rd ed. Wilmette, Mosby, 1991.

Swanson, Janice M., and Albrecht, Mary: *Community Health Nursing: Promoting the Health of Aggregates.* Philadelphia, W.B. Saunders, 1993.

White, Gladys B., (Ed.): *Ethical Dilemmas in Contemporary Nursing Practice.* Washington, D.C., American Nurses, 1992.

Wilson, Holly Skodol, and Kneisl Carol Ren: *Psychiatric Nursing,* 5th ed., Menlo Park, CA, Addison-Wesley Nursing, a division of the Benjamin Cummings Publishing Company, 1996.

Wong, Donna L., Hockenberry-Eaton, Marilyn, Wilson, David, Winkelstein, Marilyn L., and Schwartz, Patricia: *Wong's Essentials of Pediatric Nursing.* St. Louis, Mosby, 2001.

Articles and Chapters

American Academy of Pediatrics: Guidelines for home care. *Pediatrics* 74:434–436, 1995.

Callahan, Joan: Families as care-givers: limits of morality in care–giving. In Jecker, Nancy (Ed.): *Aging and Ethics: Philosophical Problems in Gerontology.* Totowa, Humana, 1992.

Collopy, Bart, Dubler, Nancy, and Zuckerman, Connie: The ethics of home care: autonomy and accommodation. *Hastings Center Report,* March/April 1990.

Fry, Sara T.: The role of caring in a theory of nursing ethics. In Holmes, Helen Bequaert and Purdy, Laura M. (Eds.): *Feminist Perspectives in Medical Ethics.* Bloomington and Indianapolis, Indiana University Press, 1992.

Jecker, Nancy: Role of intimate others. In Jecker *op. cit.*

Ladd, Rosalind Ekman, Pasquerella, Lynn, and Smith, Sheri: What to do when the end is near: Ethical issues in home health care nursing. *Public Health Nursing, 17* (2): 103-110, 2000.

Lantos, John, and Kohrman, Arthur F.: Ethical aspects of pediatric home care. *Pediatrics, 89:*920–24, 1992.

Okun, Ale: All in the family: the inequity between parental rights and home care duties. In Cassidy, Robert (Ed.): *Pediatric Ethics: From Principles to Practice.* Amsterdam, Harwood, 1996.

Stulginsky, M.M.: Nurses' home health experience. *Nursing and Health Care, 14:*405, 1993.

Professional Codes, State Regulations, and Legal Cases

American Nurses Association, Washington, D.C.: *Code for Nurses with Interpretive Statements*, 1985.

_____.: *Nursing's Social Policy Statement*, 1995.

_____.: *Standards of Home Health Nursing Practice*, 1986.

_____.: *Standards of Community Health Nursing Practice*, 1986.

Cruzan v. Director, Missouri Dept. of Health, 110 S. Ct. 2841, 1990.

Foy v. Greenblott, 141 Cal. App. 3d. 1, 13, 1983.

Jaffe v. Redmond, 518 S. Ct. 1, 1996.

Lampe v. Presbyterian Medical Center, 41 Colo. App. 465 P2d. 513, 1978.

State of Rhode Island and Providence Plantations. Department of Health. *Rules and Regulations for the Licensing of Professional Registered, Certified Registered Nurse Practitioners, Certified Registered Nurse Anesthetists, and Practical Nurses and Standards for the Approval of Basic Nursing Education Programs*, 1998.

Tarasoff v. Board of Regents of University of California, 529 P 2d 553 CA, 1976.

Tuma v. Board of Nursing, 100 Idaho 74, 593 P. 2d. 711, 1979.

Warthen v. Toms River Community Memorial Hospital, 101 N.J. 255, 501 A.2d 926 N.J., 1985.

Web Sites

http://nursingworld.org/ethics/
http://www.cybernurse.com/books/nursingethics.html

INDEX

ABOUT THE AUTHORS

Rosalind Ekman Ladd is Professor of Philosophy Emerita, Wheaton College, Norton, Massachusetts, and Lecturer in Pediatrics, Brown University Medical School. She is co-author of *Ethical Dilemmas in Pediatrics: A Case Study Approach* and editor of *Children's Rights Re-visioned: Philosophical Readings*. She has published on medical ethics, children's rights, and women's rights in health care. She serves on Ethics Committees of three hospitals in Rhode Island and has wide experience as lecturer, workshop leader, and consultant.

Lynn Pasquerella is a Professor of Philosophy at the University of Rhode Island and a Fellow in the John Hazen White Sr. Center for Ethics and Public Service. She is a graduate of Mount Holyoke College (A.B.) and Brown University (Ph.D.). Professor Pasquerella is a past recipient of the University of Rhode Island's Teaching Excellence Award and was chosen by the American Association of Higher Education and *Change* magazine as one of the "Young Leaders of the Academy." Dr. Pasquerella serves on her university's Institutional Review Board and on the Ethics Committee of Day Kimball Hospital. She has published extensively in the areas of theoretical and applied ethics, public policy, medical ethics, and the philosophy of law. Her current research focuses on the ethical and legal implications of the Human Genome Project.

Sheri Smith received her B.A. in Biology and Philosophy from Millikin University and an A.M. and Ph.D. in Philosophy from Brown University. She is a Professor of Philosophy at Rhode Island College. Professor Smith has served on the Rhode Island Department of Health's Institutional Review Board and Genetic Screening Advisory Committee. She is also a member of two hospital ethics committees and served as chair of the Ethics Advisory Committee of Roger Williams Medical Center. She has published numerous articles in the area of medical ethics and is a specialist in the field of nursing ethics. Professor Smith has also contributed as an essayist and commentator for Trinity Repertory Company's Humanities Series.

In addition to their individual work, the authors have collaborated on several articles and papers that were presented at national and international conferences:

"Infants, the Dead Donor Rule, and Organ Donation: Should the Rules Be Changed?" in *Law, Medicine and Ethics*, Volume 20, Number 3, (September 2001) and in *Proceedings of the Thirteenth World Congress on Medical Law*, Helsinki, Finland (August 2000). Pages 888-892.

"What to Do When the End is Near: Ethical Issues in Home Health Care" in *Public Health Nursing*, Volume 17, Number 2, (2000). Pages 103-110.

"In the Interest of the Fetus: Mandatory Prenatal Classes in the Workplace" in *Women and Politics*, Volume 13, Number 3/4, (1993). Pages 191–201. Reprinted in Janna Merrick, ed., *The Politics of Pregnancy:Issues in the Maternal-Fetal Relationship*. Haworth Press, 1994. Pages 191-201.

"Liability–Driven Ethics: The Impact on Hiring Practices" in *Business Ethics Quarterly*, Volume 4, Issue 3, (1994). Pages 321-333.